AF402101

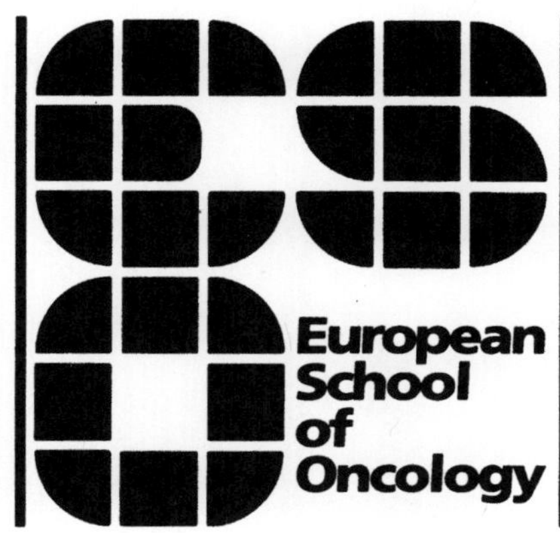

Monographs

Series Editor: U. Veronesi

The European School of Oncology gratefully acknowledges Eli Lilly and Company for an educational grant for the sponsorship of this Task Force and monograph.

M.S. Aapro (Ed.)

Innovative Antimetabolites in Solid Tumours

With 4 Figures and 18 Tables

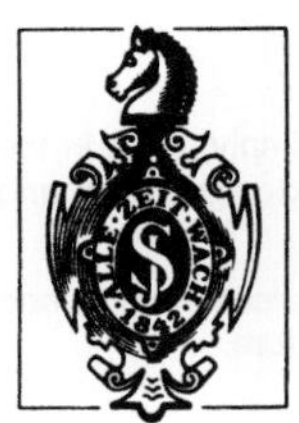

Springer-Verlag
Berlin   Heidelberg   New York
London   Paris   Tokyo
Hong Kong   Barcelona
Budapest

Matti S. Aapro

Divisione di Oncologia Medica
Istituto Europeo di Oncologia
via Ripamonti 435
20141 Milano, Italy

and

Division d'Onco-Hématologie
Hôpital Cantonal Universitaire
1211 Genève 14, Switzerland

ISBN-13: 978-3-642-79202-1   e-ISBN-13: 978-3-642-79200-7
DOI: 10.1007/978-3-642-79200-7

Library of Congress Cataloging-in-Publication Data
Innovative antimetabolites in solid tumours / M.S. Aapro (ed.)
    (ESO monographs)
Includes bibliographical references.

1. Antimetabolites--Therapeutic use.   2. Cancer--Chemotherapy.   I. Aapro, M.S. (Matti S.), 1951-.   II. Series: Monographs (European School of Oncology) [DNLM: 1. Antimetabolites--therapeutic use. 2. Neoplasms--drug therapy. QZ 267 I44 1994] RC271.A68I56 1994 616.99'4061--dc20 DNLM/DLC for Library of Congress

Typesetting: Camera ready by editor

SPIN: 10087486   19/3130 - 5 4 3 2 1 0 — Printed on acid-free paper

Foreword

The European School of Oncology came into existence to respond to a need for information, education and training in the field of the diagnosis and treatment of cancer. There are two main reasons why such an initiative was considered necessary. Firstly, the teaching of oncology requires a rigorously multidisciplinary approach which is difficult for the Universities to put into practice since their system is mainly disciplinary orientated. Secondly, the rate of technological development that impinges on the diagnosis and treatment of cancer has been so rapid that it is not an easy task for medical faculties to adapt their curricula flexibly.

With its residential courses for organ pathologies and the seminars on new techniques (laser, monoclonal antibodies, imaging techniques etc.) or on the principal therapeutic controversies (conservative or mutilating surgery, primary or adjuvant chemotherapy, radiotherapy alone or integrated), it is the ambition of the European School of Oncology to fill a cultural and scientific gap and, thereby, create a bridge between the University and Industry and between these two and daily medical practice.

One of the more recent initiatives of ESO has been the institution of permanent study groups, also called task forces, where a limited number of leading experts are invited to meet once a year with the aim of defining the state of the art and possibly reaching a consensus on future developments in specific fields of oncology.

The ESO Monograph series was designed with the specific purpose of disseminating the results of these study group meetings, and providing concise and updated reviews of the topic discussed.

It was decided to keep the layout relatively simple, in order to restrict the costs and make the monographs available in the shortest possible time, thus overcoming a common problem in medical literature: that of the material being outdated even before publication.

Umberto Veronesi
Chairman Scientific Committee
European School of Oncology

Contents

Introduction

Matti S. Aapro

Divisione di Oncologia Medica, Istituto Europeo di Oncologia, Milano, Italy, and Division d'Onco-Hématologie, Hôpital Cantonal Universitaire, Genève, Switzerland

This monograph contains a series of papers which address past and current aspects as well as recent advances in tumour therapy with antimetabolites. Almost half a century has elapsed since Farber published the demonstration of efficacy of aminopterin in childhood acute leukaemia. Maybe antimetabolites should be called the "aspirin" of oncology, as they share a long-standing history and are continuously rediscovered as a class of agents.

In this volume Zulian reviews the history of antimetabolites and also has the difficult task of discussing the value of cladribine and fludarabine in solid tumours. These agents, while playing a remarkable role in haematological malignancies, are of limited or no value in solid tumours because of enzymatic modulation and possibly dose-limiting myelosuppression. Their future role as radiation sensitizers, however, remains to be elucidated. Plunkett, Harper and Calvert give us an update on the pharmacokinetic and pharmacodynamic aspects of antimetabolites, which are yet to be fully exploited, even for a well established compound like 5-fluorouracil. While Possinger et al. and Le Chevalier present short phase II reports on gemcitabine in breast cancer and non-small cell lung cancer, Neijt and Lund and Thatcher et al. discuss various important aspects of ovarian and non-small cell lung cancer, giving a proper perspective for the development of gemcitabine in these diseases. Tonato and Mosconi review the excellent safety profile of gemcitabine, as well as that of fludarabine and cytarabine.

What should the reader remember from this publication of the European School of Oncology? Cancer therapy is a field in continuous evolution, and we should constantly go back to the historical development of our established procedures and question the validity of accepted approaches. Had we not done so, then the development of another class of active agents, the taxanes, would never have happened. How many other agents, procedures, schedules have we discarded, which should be reexamined?

Antimetabolites: Historical Perspectives

Gilbert B. Zulian

Department of Onco-Haematology, Geneva University Hospital, 1211 Geneva 14, Switzerland

Antimetabolites are structural analogues of normal metabolites that are required for cell functions and replication. As such and in order to inhibit DNA biosynthesis, they interact with enzymes in 3 different ways:
- they can substitute for a metabolite;
- they can compete with a metabolite for occupation of a catalytic site;
- they can compete with a metabolite that is acting itself as an enzyme.

Antimetabolites can be divided into 4 different categories:
- the antifolates (methotrexate, edatrexate, trimetrexate);
- the fluoropyrimidines (5-fluorouracil, ftorafur);
- the pyrimidine analogues (cytarabine, 5-azacytidine, gemcitabine);
- the purine analogues (6-thioguanine, 6-mercaptopurine, deoxycoformycin, fludarabine, cladribine).

Their common target of toxicity is the DNA which they reach via different pathways, thereby inducing a distinct spectrum of clinical activity. These agents cover not only the major part of medical oncology and anticancer therapy but also some purely immunological areas. This report will focus on the best known and most widely utilised antimetabolites with emphasis on their mechanism of action and toxicities (Tables 1 and 2).

Antifolates

Methotrexate

The history of antimetabolites started shortly after the second World War with the 4-amino analogue of folic acid, aminopterin, which was shown in 1948 to be active against some childhood leukaemias [1]. Several analogues of this compound were then synthesized, among which methotrexate (MTX) emerged as the most useful and still is until now [2,3]. MTX, the 4-amino, 10-methyl analogue of aminopterin, is an inhibitor of the enzyme dihydrofolate reduc-

Table 1. Antimetabolites with definite activity in the management of solid tumours

Methotrexate (folic acid antagonist)	breast head and neck osteosarcoma choriocarcinoma
5-fluorouracil (fluoropyrimidine)	colon rectum breast head and neck stomach pancreas (?)
Gemcitabine (deoxycytidine analogue)	lung (?)

Table 2. Main toxicities of antimetabolites

	BM	M	K	L	N	P	C	G	HF	S
Methotrexate	x	x	x	x	x	x				
5-fluorouracil	x	x			x			x	x	x
Cytarabine	x	x			x			x	x	
Gemcitabine	x	x								x
6-mercaptopurine	x	x		x				x		
6-thioguanine	x	x		(x)				x		
Deoxycoformycin	x		x	x	x					
Fludarabine	x				x					
Cladribine	x		x		x					

BM = bone marrow; M = mucosa; K = kidney; L = liver; N = neurological; P = pulmonary; C = cardiac; G = gut;
HF= hand-foot syndrome; S = skin

tase (DHFR), and this interaction results in the depletion of as much as 50% to 60% of the intracellular pool of folate [4]. More recently, MTX was shown to be polyglutamated, leading to the inhibition of enzymes such as transformylases and thymidylate synthetase, and to further inhibition of DHFR [5]. MTX is a cell-cycle specific agent, which means that cells have to be in the S-phase in order to be appropriately damaged by this agent. Furthermore, MTX cytotoxicity is highly dependent upon drug concentration and duration of exposure of the drug in the cell [3]. Resistance to MTX is mediated by an increase in DHFR gene [6], DHFR protein expression [7], alteration of MTX transport mechanisms and a decrease in polyglutamation [3]. The side-effects of MTX include myelosuppression, mucositis, nephrotoxicity, hepatotoxicity, neurotoxicity and pneumonitis. Pulmonary fibrosis has also been described when MTX is given chronically at low doses. MTX toxicity can markedly increase in the case of body fluid collection, so-called "third space", since the excretion will be prolonged due to continuous release. MTX is excreted via the kidneys and this can be inhibited by non-steroidal anti-inflammatory drugs, penicillins and cephalosporins. Thanks to the appropriate use of folinic acid, the side-effects of MTX can be totally avoided in practice and this has permitted to give very high doses that would have otherwise been lethal.

MTX has a wide field of application in medical oncology including leukaemia and lymphoma, breast cancer, head and neck cancer, osteogenic sarcoma and choriocarcinoma, the latter being the first metastatic solid tumour cured by chemotherapy [8]. MTX is also used as an immunomodulator, for example in psoriasis, rheumatoid arthritis and graft-versus-host disease. It can even be used as an adjuvant to antibiotics in bacterial and plasmodial infections and parasitic infections in AIDS. Orally, MTX is given in dosages up to 25 mg/m^2 because of its poor bioavailability. MTX is generally administered intravenously and at very high doses providing folinic acid rescue is also given. Intrathecal injection is routinely used therapeutically or prophylactically in leukaemias and high-grade lymphomas and in the case of carcinomatous meningitis. The intra-arterial, pleural, pericardial and peritoneal routes have also been used.

Other Antifolates

New antifolates have been developed, among which trimetrexate [9], edatrexate [10], pyritrexim [11], PT523 [12], D1694 [13], CB3717 [14] and lometrexol [15]. These agents have not yet found standard clinical applications.

Fluoropyrimidines

5-Fluorouracil

5-Fluorouracil (5-FU) is a synthetic compound [16] with 3 active metabolites:

- 5-fluoro-deoxyuridine monophosphate (5-FdUMP), which is an inhibitor of thymidylate synthetase (TS) and thereby of DNA biosynthesis [17];
- fluorouridine triphosphate (FUTP), which is incorporated into RNA;
- fluoro-deoxyuridine triphosphate (FdUTP), which is directly incorporated into DNA [18].

In order to form the 5-FdUMP-TS complex, the presence of intracellular reduced folate acting as a cofactor is necessary [19]. Concomitant administration of folinic acid (FA) increases the cytotoxicity of 5-FU [20] as well as prior administration of MTX [21]. Synergism has also been suggested with dipyridamole [22] and alpha-interferon [23]. Resistance is mediated through deletion of activating key enzymes or from increase in TS synthesis [24]. The side-effects of 5-FU include myelosuppression, mucositis, diarrhoea, the hand-foot syndrome, dermatitis, neurotoxicity, vascular toxicity and cardiotoxicity. The catabolism of 5-FU is strongly dependent on dihydropyrimidine dehydrogenase (DPD) and deficiency of this enzyme can lead to a dramatic increase in its toxicity [25]. Clinical applications cover colorectal cancer, head and neck cancer, breast cancer, gastric and pancreatic cancer and ovarian cancer. 5-FU has only 25% bioavailabilty and oral administration is therefore not recommendable. It is usually given intravenously but can also be infused intra-arterially and intraperitoneally or even topically.

Other Fluoropyrimidines

5-Fluoro-2-deoxyuridine (FUdR) and 1-2-tetrahydrofuranyl-5-fluorouracil (ftorafur) are two other fluoropyrimidines still under investigation for clinical use.

Pyrimidine (Cytidine) Analogues (Fig. 1)

Cytarabine

Cytarabine or cytosine arabinoside was isolated from the sponge Cryptothetya crypta and is an analogue of 2'deoxycytidine (pyrimidine nucleotide). Cytarabine is phosphorylated to its active metabolite arabinoside-cytosine-triphosphate (ara-CTP) by a 3-step enzymatic reaction with deoxycytidine kinase (dCTk), deoxycytidylate kinase and nucleoside diphosphate kinase. Ara-CTP inhibits DNA polymerase and is also incorporated into DNA [26]. This results in the initiation of apoptosis or programmed cell death. Cytarabine cytotoxicity is highly cell-cycle specific and only cells in the S-phase are actively killed. Inactivation of cytarabine is dependent upon cytidine deaminase and resistance is caused either by dCTk deficiency or by inadequate transport. The side-effects of cytarabine include myelosuppression, mucositis, nausea, vomiting, conjunctivitis, hand-foot syndrome and neurotoxicity. Interaction with other cytotoxic drugs such as MTX, cyclophosphamide, etoposide, carmustine and cisplatin can enhance their toxicity. Enhancement of cytarabine cytotoxicity occurs with the concomitant administration of tetrahydrouridine or hydroxyurea [27]. Cytarabine is mainly used in acute leukaemias and refractory lymphomas and can be given at very high doses [28]. The route of administration can be intravenous, subcutaneous or intrathecal. Cytarabine cannot be given orally because of the high concentration of cytidine deaminase in the gut.

5-Azacytidine

5-Azacytidine is a cytidine analogue that is phosphorylated by uridine-cytidine kinase to 5-azacytidine-triphosphate [29]. 5-Azacytidine appears useful only in the management of acute leukaemia with side-effects including myelosuppression, nausea and vomiting, liver toxicity, myalgias, skin rash and pruritus.

Gemcitabine

Gemcitabine is an analogue of deoxycytidine and must be phosphorylated to difluoro-deoxycytidine-triphosphate in order to inhibit DNA polymerase. Gemcitabine is myelosuppressive and causes mucositis as well as dermatitis while being active against leukaemias [30] and various solid tumours. The present ESO monograph contains several important reports concerning this promising new drug.

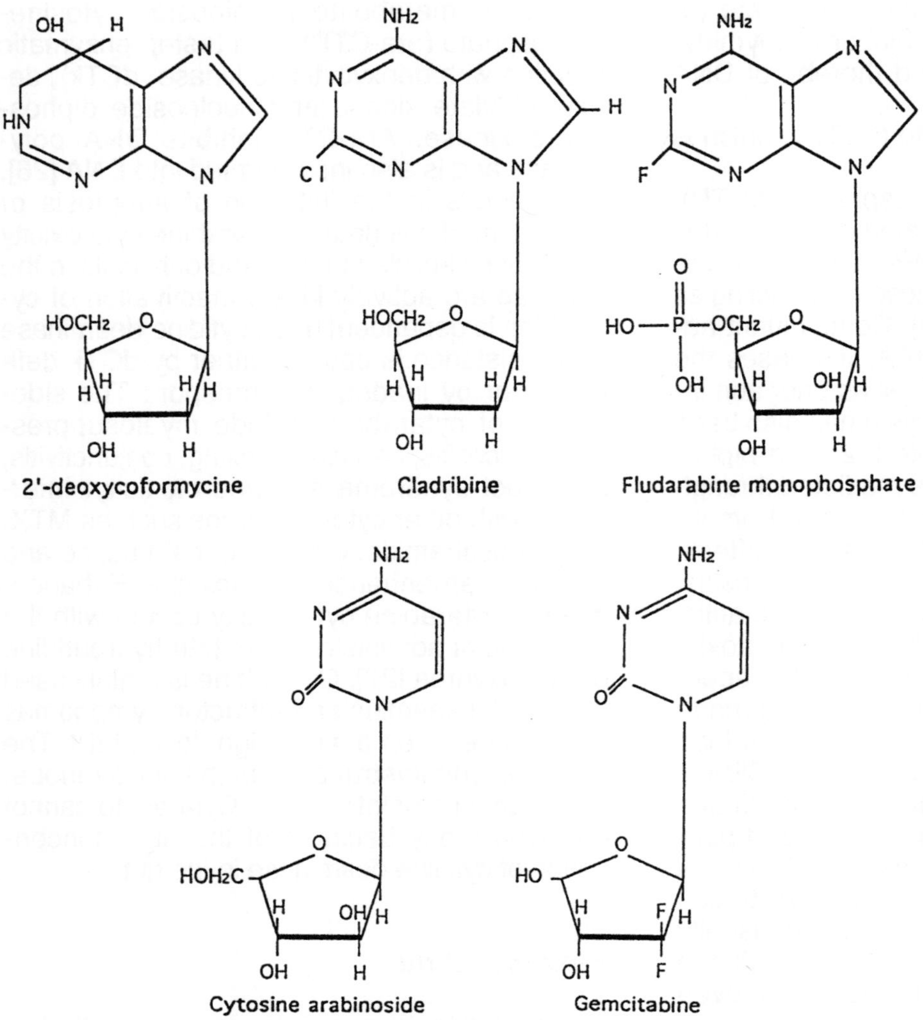

Fig. 1. Structure of purine and pyrimidine analogues

Purine Analogues

6-Mercaptopurine and 6-Thioguanine

6-Mercaptopurine (6-MP) and 6-thioguanine (6-TG) are the respective analogues of hypoxanthine and guanine. They are activated by hypoxanthine-guanine-phosphoribosyl-transferase and inhibit purine synthesis in synergy with MTX [31]. The cytotoxicity of 6-TG can be increased by concomitant administration of allopurinol [32]. 6-MP is used as maintenance therapy in acute lymphoblastic leukaemia while 6-TG is used for remission or maintenance of acute myeloblastic leukaemia. Both compounds are myelosuppressive and can induce nausea, vomiting, stomatitis and hepatotoxicity with cholestatic jaundice. Administration is via the oral route despite an erratic bioavailability which can vary depending on food or medication (e.g. cotrimoxazole). Besides their antileukaemic activity, these agents and their parent compound azathioprine are potent immunosuppressors frequently prescribed in case of rheumatoid arthritis, Crohn's disease, ulcerative colitis and transplant rejection.

Deoxycoformycin

Deoxycoformycin (DCF) was isolated from *Streptomyces antibioticus* and is a potent inhibitor of adenosine deaminase (ADA), an enzyme implicated in the catabolism of purine nucleotides [33]. Genetic ADA deficiency is responsible for the SCID (severe combined immune deficiency) syndrome in which both the number and the function of lymphocytes are dramatically decreased. Inhibition of ADA results in the intracellular accumulation of deoxyadenosine triphosphate (dATP) and ultimately cell death. DCF is myelosuppressive, nephrotoxic, hepatotoxic and neurotoxic and specifically used intravenously in the treatment of hairy cell leukaemia [34].

Fludarabine

Several compounds have been derived from cytarabine among which 9-ß-arabinofuranosyladenine (ara-A). Ara-A is rapidly degraded by ADA and poorly soluble. Fluorination of Ara-A has made the molecule resistant to ADA and phosphorylation has increased its solubility, thus producing a new adenosine analogue, fludarabine monophosphate (FAMP) [35]. FAMP is phosphorylated in the cell to fludarabine triphosphate by dCTK and incorporated into DNA, blocking its biosynthesis and initiating apoptosis [36]. In contrast to many other antimetabolites, FAMP is active in resting non-dividing cells. It is administered intravenously in leukaemia and lymphoma. The side-effects include myelosuppression, neuropathy and neurotoxicity. Synergy with cytarabine has been shown in leukaemia [37] and a phase III randomised study is in progress within the EORTC on the primary treatment of advanced low-grade non-Hodgkin's lymphoma.

Cladribine

Cladribine (CDA) is another adenosine analogue resistant to deamination by ADA because of chlorulation [38]. CDA is phosphorylated to 2-chloro-deoxy-adenosine-triphosphate by dCTk. CDA is active in resting non-dividing cells and induces apoptosis after incorporation into DNA [36]. Resistance to CDA appears to be mediated by the biological activity of 5'-nucleotidase and sensitivity by the total amount of dCTk in the cell [39]. Side-effects are myelosuppression, peripheral neuropathy and nephrotoxicity. CDA is used in lymphoma and leukaemia, mainly hairy cell leukaemia for which FDA approval has been granted. The route of administration is usually intravenous but the subcutaneous and oral routes are also used [40].

Summary

Antimetabolites have determined the history of medical oncology since the very early days. Their mechanism of action is particularly astute as they take advantage of normal metabolites through physiological pathways. They are active agents in most areas of cancer therapy but their wide spectrum of toxicity still indicates a rather poor selectivity. Continuously improving the knowledge of their mechanisms of action should result in better treatment, especially in the field of solid tumours which represent the vast majority of malignancies in our daily practice.

REFERENCES

1   Farber S, Diamond LK, Mercer RD et al: Temporary remissions in acute leukemia in children produced by folic acid antagonist, 4-aminopteroyl-glutamic acid (aminopterin). N Engl J Med 1948 (238):787-793

2   Goldin A: Preclinical methodology for the selection of anticancer agents. In: Bush H (ed) Methods in Cancer Research, Vol IV. Academic Press, New York 1968, pp 193-254

3   Bertino JR: Ode to methotrexate. J Clin Oncol 1993 (11):5-14

4   Osborne MJ, Freeman M, Huennekens FM: Inhibition of dihydrofolic reductase by aminopterin and ame-nothopterin. Proc Soc Exp Biol Med 1958 (97):429-431

5   Chabner BA, Allegra CA, Curt GA et al: Polygluta-mation of methotrexate. Is methotrexate a prodrug? J Clin Invest 1985 (76):907-912

6   Alt FW, Kellems RE, Bertino JR et al: Selective multiplication of dihydrofolate reductase genes in methotrexate resistant variants of cultured murine cells. J Biol Chem 1978 (253):1357-1370

7   Fischer GA: Increased levels of folic acid reductase as a mechanism of resistance to methopterin in leukemic cells. Biochem Pharmacol 1961 (7):75-77

8   Li MC, Hertz R, Spencer DB: Effect of methotrexate therapy upon choriocarcinoma and chorioadenoma. Proc Soc Exp Biol Med 1956 (93):361-366

9   Robert F: Trimetrexate as a single agent in patients with advanced head and neck cancer. Semin Oncol 1988 (15):22-26

10 Sirotnak FM, DeGraw JI, Maccio DM et al: New folate analogs of the 10-deaza-aminopterin series. Basis for structural design and biochemical and pharma-cologic properties. Cancer Chemother Pharmacol 1984 (12):13-25

11 Feun LG, Gonzalez R, Savaraj N et al: Phase II trial of pyritrexim in metastatic melanoma using intermittent, low-dose administration. J Clin Oncol 1991 (9):464-467

12 Rosowsky A, Bader H, Frei E III: In vitro and in vivo antitumor activity of N^α(4-amino-4deoxypteroyl)-N^α-hemi-phthaloyl-L-ornithine (PT523), a potent side chain modified aminopterin analog that cannot form polyglutamates. Proc Am Assoc Cancer Res 1991 (32):325 (abstract)

13 Jackman AL, Taylor GA, Gibson W et al: ICI D1694, a quinazoline antifolate thymidylate synthase inhibitor that is a potent inhibitor of L1210 tumor cell growth in vitro and in vivo. A new agent for clinical study. Cancer Res 1992 (51):5579-5586

14 Calvert AH, Newell DR, Jackman AL et al: Recent preclinical and clinical studies with the thymidylate synthase inhibitor N^{10}-propargyl-5,8-dideazofolic acid (CB3717). NCI Monograph 1987 (5):213-218

15 Beardsley GP, Moroson BA, Taylor EC et al: A new folate antimetabolite, 5-10-dideaza-5,6,7,8-tetra-hydrofolate is a potent inhibitor of de novo purine synthesis. J Biol Chem 1989 (264):328-333

16 Heidelberger C, Chandhari NK, Danenberg P et al: Fluorinated pyrimidines. A new class of tumor inhibitory compounds. Nature 1957 (179):663-666

17 Lockshin A, Danenberg PV: Biochemical factors affecting the tightness of 5-fluorodeoxyuridylate binding to human thymidilate synthetase. Biochem Pharmacol 1981 (30):247-257

18 Houghton JA, Maroda SJ, Philips JO, Houghton PJ: Biochemical determinants of responsiveness to 5-fluorouracil and its derivatives in xenografts of human adenocarcinomas in mice. Cancer Res 1981 (41):144-149

19 Evans RM, Laskin JD, Hakala MT: Effect of excess folates and deoxyinosine on the activity and site of action of 5-fluorouracil. Cancer Res 1981 (441):3288

20 Keyomarski K, Moran RG: Folinic acid augmentation of the effects of fluoropyrimidines on murine and human leukemic cells. Cancer Res 1986 (46):5229-5235

21 Cadman EC, Heimer R, Davis L: Enhanced 5-fluorouracil nucleotide formation following metho-trexate. Biochemical explanation for drug syner-gism. Science 1979 (205):1135-1137

22 Grem JL, Fischer PH: Enhancement of 5-fluoro-uracil's anticancer activity by dipyridamole. Pharmac Ther 1989 (40):349-371

23 Miyoshi T, Ogawa S, Kanamori T et al: Interferon potentiates cytotoxic effects of 5-fluorouracil on cell proliferation of established human cell lines originating from neoplastic tissues. Cancer Lett 1983 (17):239-247

24 Jenh GH, Geyer PK, Baskin F et al: Thymidilate synthase gene amplifiation in fluorodeoxyuridine-resistant mouse cell lines. Mol Pharmacol 1985 (28):80-85

25 Houyau P, Gay C, Chatelut E et al: Severe fluoro-uracil toxicity in a patient with dihydropyrimidine dehydrogenase deficiency. JNCI 1993 (85):1602-1603

26 Inagati A, Nakamera T, Wakinosaka G: Studies of the mechanism of action of 1-beta-D-arabino-furanosycytosine as an inhibitor of DNA synthesis in human leukemic leukocytes. Cancer Res 1969 (29):2169-2176

27 Schilsky RL, Williams SF, Ultmann JE, Watson S: Sequential hydroxyurea-cytarabine chemotherapy for refractory non-Hodgkin's lymphoma. J Clin Oncol 1987 (5):419-425

28 Plunkett W, Liliemark JO, Adams TM et al: Saturation of 1-beta-D-arabinofuranosylcytosine-5'-triphosphate accumulation in leukemia cells during high dose 1-beta-D-arabinofuranosylcytosine thera-py. Cancer Res 1987 (47):3005-3011

29 Glover AB, Leyland-Jones BR, Chun HG, Davies B, Hoth DF: Azacytidine: 10 years later. Cancer Treat Rep 1987 (71):737-746

30 Grunewald R, Kantarjian H, Faucher K, Tarassoff P, Plunkett W: Gemcitabine in leukemia: a phase I clinical, plasma and cellular pharmacology study. J Clin Oncol 1992 (10):406-413

31 Balis FM, Holcenberg JS, Zimm S et al: The effect of methotrexate on the bioavailability of oral 6-mercaptopurine. Clin Pharmacol Ther 1987 (41):384-387

32 Coffey JJ, White CA, Lesk AB et al: Effect of allopu-rinol on the pharmacokinetics of 6-mercaptopurine in cancer patients. Cancer Res 1972 (32):1283-1289

33 Glazer RI: Adenosine deaminase inhibitors: their role in chemotherapy and immmunosuppression. Cancer Chemother Pharmacol 1980 (4):227-235

34 Kraut EH, Bouroncle BA, Grever MR: Pentostatin in the treatment of advanced hairy cell leukemia. J Clin Oncol 1989 (7):168-172

35 Plunkett W, Huang P, Gandhi V: Metabolism and action of fludarabine phosphate. Semin Oncol 1990 (17):3-17

36 Robertson LE, Chubb S, Meyn RE et al: Induction of apoptotic cell death in chronic lymphocytic leukemia by 2-chloro-2'-deoxyadenosine and 9-ß-D-arabinosyl-2-fluoroadenine. Blood 1993 (81):143-150

37 Gandhi V, Estey E, Keating MJ, Plunkett W: Fludarabine potentiates metabolism of cytarabine in patients with acute myelogenous leukemia during therapy. J Clin Oncol 1993 (11):116-124

38 Beutler E: Cladribine (2-chlorodeoxyadenosine). Lancet 1992 (340):952-956

39 Kawasaki K, Carrera CJ, Piro LD et al: Relationship of deoxycytidine kinase and cytoplasmic 5'-nucleotidase to the chemotherapeutic efficacy of 2-chlorodeoxyadenosine. Blood 1993 (81):597-601

40 Liliemark J, Albertioni F, Hassan M, Juliusson G: On the bioavailability of oral and subcutaneous 2-chloro-2'-deoxyadenosine in humans. Alternative routes of administration. J Clin Oncol 1992 (10): 1514-1518

Preclinical Characteristics of Cytarabine, Gemcitabine, Fludarabine and Cladribine: Relevance for Clinical Studies

William Plunkett

Section of Cellular and Molecular Pharmacology, The University of Texas M.D. Anderson Cancer Center, 1515 Holcombe Boulevard, Houston, Texas 77030, USA

Understanding the pharmacokinetics of anti-cancer drugs is essential to the optimal design of therapeutic regimes. By extension, a knowledge of cellular metabolism and the mechanisms by which metabolites exert their activities also provides valuable information for strategies combining agents or modalities. Nucleoside antimetabolites comprise one of the most effective classes of drugs for the treatment of cancer and viral diseases. Universally, nucleoside analogues are active only after entry into the cell and phosphorylation to nucleotide derivatives, generally the corresponding triphosphates. Their biological activity is due to the fact that most nucleoside analogues are targeted at DNA synthesis, an essential function both for cellular replication and for the repair of DNA damage that may be caused by other agents.

Cytarabine has long been the paradigm of nucleoside antimetabolites. It is the single most effective agent in adult acute leukaemias and exhibits activity in other leukaemias and lymphomas [1,2]. Unfortunately, numerous trials in solid tumours have indicated that its activity is confined to the haematological malignancies.

Nevertheless, several new nucleoside antimetabolites which have unique spectra of clinical activity, gemcitabine, fludarabine, and cladribine, have recently been developed. Unlike cytarabine, these drugs exhibit multiple mechanisms of action, which suggests that they may have clinical potential alone and in combinations that surpass that of cytarabine. This chapter will review and compare the pharmacology and mechanisms of action of these agents with a goal of formulating a rationale for their optimal use in combination with other drugs and radiotherapy.

The structures of cytarabine, gemcitabine, fludarabine and cladribine are shown in Figure 1. The major locus of action of all nucleosides is at DNA synthesis. It is not surprising, therefore, that three of the drugs have alterations at the 2'-carbon, the site on nucleosides at which DNA metabolising enzymes discriminate. Cytarabine and fludarabine are both arabinosyl nucleosides, whereas gemcitabine possesses geminal fluorines, from whence it derives its name [3]. Earlier studies demonstrated that vidarabine (arabinosyladenine) was inactive in human leukaemias primarily because of

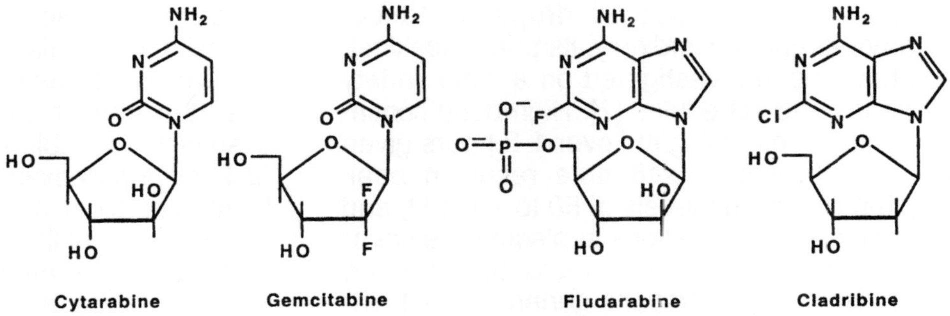

Fig. 1. Chemical structures of nucleoside analogues

Table 1. Clinical pharmacology of nucleoside analogues

Drug	Dose mg/m^2	Infusion duration (hr)	C_{max} µM	C_{ss} µM	Elimination t1/2 (hr)	Clearance
Cytarabine	3,000	1-3	50-100	-	0.2	metabolic
	500	2	10	-	0.2	
	1,500	24	-	1-3	-	
	200	24	-	0.05	-	
Gemcitabine	800	0.5	40	-	0.15	metabolic
	1,200-4,800	2-8		25	-	
Fludarabine	20-30	0.5	1-3	-	10-30	renal
	30*	24	-	7	-	
Cladribine	5.6	2	0.2	0.03-0.020	8	renal
	1-5.6	24	-		-	

* loading bolus followed by continuous infusion

metabolic clearance by adenosine deaminase, and that its relative insolubility curtailed efforts to circumvent this inactivation by increasing the dose [4]. Because it was known that a halogen on the 2-carbon of adenine protected adenine nucleosides from deamination, this modification of vidarabine was made to create fludarabine, and the 5'-phosphate was added to enhance the solubility of the compound. Thus, fludarabine is formulated as a nucleotide. Cladribine is the 2-chloro derivative of deoxyadenosine, and like fludarabine, this substitution confers resistance to inactivation by adenosine deaminase [6].

Pharmacology

An overview of the general pharmacokinetic characteristics of each nucleoside antimetabolite after intravenous administration is presented in Table 1. Cytarabine is one of the most thoroughly studied drugs in cancer chemotherapy. Accordingly, its pharmacokinetics have been investigated on a wide variety of doses and schedules [7]. High-dose continuous infusions of 3 g/m^2 over 1-3 hours given on an intermittent schedule result in peak plasma cytarabine levels of 50 to 100 µM, and cytarabine concentrations in plasma are linear over a wide range of dose rates [8]. However, the plasma concentrations generated by high-dose cytarabine regimens are greatly in excess of those which saturate the rate of cytarabine phosphorylation (10 µM) [9]. Therefore, recent studies have utilised somewhat lower dose rates, 0.25- 0.5 mg/m^2/h, characterised as intermediate-dose cytarabine, to maximize the accumulation of active cytarabine triphosphate in leukaemia cells while reducing toxicity [10]. Continuous infusions of either high-dose (1.5 mg/m^2 per day) or conventional-dose cytarabine (100-200 mg/m^2 per day) also produce steady-state cytarabine levels proportional to the dose rate [11]. Following infusion, cytarabine is cleared by deamination to the inactive compound, arabinosyluracil, with a terminal half-life of less than 20 min [12]. Interestingly, after high-dose infusions, a more prolonged terminal elimination phase is observed [13]. Because greater concentrations of cytarabine phosphate are accumulated in tissues after high-dose regimens, it is possible that the apparent slower elimination is due to continued release of cytarabine from tissues after dephosphorylation of the high cellular concentrations of cytarabine nucleotide that accumulate. Gemcitabine is also an excellent substrate for deoxycytidine deaminase; it is cleared rapidly after the end of infusions [14,15]. As is the case with cytarabine, the deamination product (2',2'-difluorodeoxyuridine) does not appear to have biological activity [16]. Most phase II studies have utilised 30-min infusions of 800 mg/m^2, a dose rate which generates 40 to 50 µM gemcitabine in plasma [14]. Again, as was the case with cytarabine, this concentration exceeds the level that can be utilised by deoxycytidine kinase and thus limits the accumulation of active gemcitabine nucleotides in mononuclear cells and leukaemia blasts [14,17,18]. Additional trials were conducted with the goal of maximizing the accumulation of gemcitabine nucleotides in leukaemia cells by infusing gemcitabine at a rate (600 mg/m^2/h) that would achieve 20 µM gemcitabine plasma levels [15,18]. This dose rate produced a median steady-state value of 25 µM gemcitabine, and could be continued safely for 8 hours in patients with relapsed acute leukaemia. Associated investigations demonstrated that gemcitabine triphosphate accumulation continued at linear rates in leukaemia blasts for the duration of these infusions.

Fludarabine is most frequently administered in daily 30-min infusions of 20 to 30 mg/m^2 in current therapeutic use [19]. Because fludarabine is rapidly and quantitatively dephosphorylated to the nucleoside arabinosyl-2-fluoroadenine (F-ara-A) upon intravenous infusion, it has not been possible to study the parent nucleotide. Thus the investigations of the pharmacokinetics of fludarabine have all been based on studies of the nucleoside metabolite, which for purposes of simplicity will be considered synonymous with the parent drug. Plasma levels of fludarabine of 1 to 3 µM are achieved by the end of a 30-min infusion of 18-30 mg/m^2 [20,21]. In contrast to cytarabine and gemcitabine, fludarabine is cleared principally by renal excretion [22]. Most studies utilising ultraviolet detection have described a terminal half-life of elimination of about 10 hours, whereas a more sensitive fluorescence assay has recently indicated a terminal half-life of 30 hours [23]. A study in paediatric patients of a loading bolus of fludarabine followed by continuous infusion resulted in 7 µM fludarabine at steady-state [24].

The pharmacokinetics of cladribine have been studied after both intermittent short-term administration and continuous infusions [25,26]. Because the typical dose of cladribine is substantially less than that of fludarabine, it is not surprising that the peak plasma concentration is lower than that of fludarabine. Like fludarabine, cladribine is resistant to catabolism; elimination is predominantly via the renal route with a terminal half-life of 8 hours. When administered as a continuous infusion, a proportionality was observed between dose rate and steady-state concentrations of cladribine.

Mechanisms of Action

It is likely that all of the nucleoside antimetabolites enter the cell by a low-specificity, high-capacity facilitated transport mechanism. For biological activity, each drug must be metabolised to the corresponding nucleotide derivatives, among which the triphosphate is generally the active form. The common essential step in the metabolism of each nucleoside involves phosphorylation to the monophosphate by deoxycytidine kinase [27-30]. This initial phosphorylation is rate limiting in the metabolism of all the nucleosides to the respective triphosphates except for cladribine. Studies in cell culture and *in vitro* investigations in fresh human leukaemia cells demonstrated that the cladribine monophosphate accumulated to the highest concentrations of all nucleotide derivatives [31]. This suggests that, as is the case with zidovudine, phosphorylation of cladribine monophosphate is rate limiting for formation of the active triphosphate.

Phosphorylation

Deoxycytidine kinase exhibits more than a 100-fold range in affinity (Km) for the nucleoside antimetabolites (Table 2). Gemcitabine appears to be the best substrate, whereas the enzyme has a relatively low affinity for fludarabine [29,30,32]. This is important when considering the scheduling of these drugs in combinations. For instance, there is actually a rise in the fludarabine concentration in plasma during cytarabine infusion [33]. This is consistent with the hypothesis that, because of its greater affinity for cytarabine, deoxycytidine kinase phosphorylates ara-C in preference to fludarabine. Fludarabine in the cell is not phosphorylated and effluxes to the blood during cytarabine infusion, thus altering fludarabine pharmacokinetics.

Table 2. Comparison of metabolism and mechanisms of action of nucleoside analogues

Site of action	Cytarabine	Gemcitabine	Fludarabine	Cladribine
Km for deoxycytidine kinase	10	2	200-400	40
Ribonucleotide reductase inhibition	no	yes	yes	yes
t1/2 of triphosphate elimination	rapid	slow*	slow	rapid
DNA termination	weak	strong**	strong	weak
Excision for DNA	yes	resistant	resistant	?
Inhibits DNA ligation	weak	?	potent	?
Self-potentiation	none	multiple	some	some

*   Elimination of gemcitabine triphosphate is concentration dependent; monophasic at cellular concentrations <100 µM, but biphasic at higher concentrations with a prolonged terminal elimination rate
**   Gemcitabine is incorporated predominantly in the penultimate position in DNA primer elongation assays

Ribonucleotide Reductase

The major source of deoxynucleotides which are required for DNA synthesis and repair is ribonucleotide reductase. The triphosphates of both fludarabine and cladribine are effective inhibitors of ribonucleotide reductase and bring about a decrease in cellular deoxynucleotides [34,35] (Table 2). It is assumed that the mechanism of this inhibition involves the interaction of the analogue triphosphates with the global allosteric inhibitory site on the enzyme. Gemcitabine appears to inhibit ribonucleotide reductase by a different mechanism. The diphosphate of gemcitabine serves as an inhibitory alternative substrate, inhibiting the enzyme in a mechanism-based fashion [36,37]. The details of this activity remain to be elucidated. In contrast, the nucleotides of cytarabine do not appear to affect the activity of ribonucleotide reductase [38].

Triphosphate Elimination

Because the triphosphate of each nucleotide analogue is the proximal active metabolite, its residence time in the cell is likely to be directly related to the potency of its cytoxicity. Although heterogeneity in the half-life of elimination is the hallmark of nucleotides among both cell lines and fresh human leukaemia cells, there is an obvious difference in the general ability of cells to retain the triphosphates of different nucleosides. For instance, after infusion of cytarabine its triphosphate is eliminated from human leukaemia cells with a median half-life of 2-3 hours with monophasic kinetics [39] (Table 2). In contrast, the triphosphates of both fludarabine and gemcitabine are eliminated relatively slowly. Interestingly, gemcitabine triphosphate exhibits a concentration-dependent elimination which is biphasic with an exceedingly long terminal half-life when the concentration of triphosphate exceeds 100 µM in cells in culture and in leukaemia cells during therapy [15,16,40]. Elimination of cladribine triphosphate has been studied only in cells in culture, in which it has a relatively brief retention after parent nucleoside is removed [31]. These properties have implications for the dose schedules upon which these drugs might be administered to achieve and maintain maximal concentration of the active triphosphate metabolites. For instance, cytarabine and cladribine might best be administered as continuous infusions or a frequent intermittent schedule, whereas daily administration of fludarabine and gemcitabine could be adequate to maintain therapeutic levels of triphosphate in target cells.

DNA Incorporation

The triphosphates of each nucleoside antimetabolite do not directly inhibit DNA polymerases. Rather, they have Km values for incorporation that are similar to those of the competing deoxynucleotides; therefore, they must be considered relatively good substrates for incorporation into DNA. With the exception of inhibition of ribonucleotide reductase as mentioned above, the principal activity of the nucleoside analogues occurs after their incorporation into DNA. Thus it appears that relative to the ability of an incorporated nucleotide analogue to inhibit the subsequent addition of deoxynucleotides may be a measure of the potency of each drug. Although direct comparisons of this property have not yet been made, the relative ability of an analogue to terminate a DNA strand may serve as a surrogate measurement of this activity (Table 2). In this sense it is known that most of the cytarabine nucleotide incorporated into DNA in whole cells resides internally in the DNA strands, suggesting that it is a weak DNA chain terminator [41]. Model systems have demonstrated that cladribine is a fair substrate for the addition of deoxynucleotides by purified human DNA polymerases [42], although this property has not been evaluated in intact cells. In contrast, greater than 95% of the fludarabine nucleotide incorporated into the DNA of intact cells is located at the terminus, indicating that it is an effective DNA chain terminator [43]. As an interesting hybrid, studies in whole cells demonstrate that gemcitabine nucleotide is mainly internal in DNA recovered from whole cells [44]. Model systems, however, demonstrated that the triphosphate of this drug has the unique property of being incorporated, permitting the DNA polymerase to incorporate a single additional deoxynucleotide, and then the enzyme is greatly inhibited in further nucleotide incorporation [44]. As such, gemcitabine nucleotide may serve as a masked nucleotide analogue in that it exerts its chain terminating activity from a position somewhat distant from the actual DNA terminus.

Excision from DNA

It is now generally appreciated that several mammalian DNA polymerases possess exonuclease activities which degrade one strand of the DNA duplex in the 3' to 5' direction. These exonucleases are thought to function as proof-reading activities that remove mismatched base pairs once the polymerising portion of the DNA polymerase perceives such an error. This signal is probably transmitted as a change in the configuration of the template-primer in the polymerisation active site. Such a signal might also be generated by the steric shift produced once a nucleotide analogue has been incorporated in place of the deoxynucleotide. If we assume that the cytotoxic activity of a nucleotide analogue is derived from its ability to inhibit further DNA synthesis once it has been incorporated into the growing DNA strand, and that the exonuclease activities associated with the DNA polymerases have the capability of removing the nucleotide analogue to permit the resumption of DNA synthesis, then the efficiency of analogue removal by the exonuclease would be an indicator of the relative resistance of the cell to inhibition by any particular nucleotide antimetabolite. As of yet, only DNA polymerase epsilon has been evaluated for the ability of its associated 3' → 5' exonuclease to remove nucleotide analogues from DNA termini. Cytarabine nucleotide was excised at roughly one third the rate of deoxynucleotides, and eventually all of the drug containing DNA was degraded [44]. In contrast, gemcitabine nucleotide was relatively resistant to excision from the 3'-terminus [44]. Furthermore, when gemcitabine nucleotide was placed one nucleotide from the 3'-terminus, the position in which it resides predominantly in model DNA synthesis systems, it was essentially resistant to excision. This further indicated that the masked feature of its incorporation at the penultimate position in a growing DNA strand may play an important role in gemcitabine's action. Fludarabine is an effective DNA chain terminator, but studies demonstrate that the exonuclease of DNA polymerase epsilon is unable to remove it [43]. In addition, recent findings indicate that in the process of trying to remove fludarabine nucleotide, both the exonuclease and DNA polymerising activities of the enzyme may be inactivated [45]. Thus, the newer nucleotide antimetabolites exhibit properties which make them potentially more effective inhibitors of DNA replication and repair than does cytarabine.

DNA Ligation

The joining of two single strands of DNA annealed in adjacent positions on a DNA template is the function of DNA ligase I. This activity is an essential natural function in DNA replication and repair. Because the nucleotide antimetabolites reside at the 3'-end of an elongating strand of DNA, and to relative extents inhibit further elongation, it may be of importance to know the consequences of drug incorporation on DNA ligase I activity. This has been evaluated for cytarabine nucleotide which was found to be a possible but suboptimal substrate for ligation [46]. In contrast, when fludarabine nucleotide was placed at the 3'-terminus of a piece of DNA, it strongly inhibited joining of that end with an adjacent piece of DNA [47]. Furthermore, at clinically achievable concentrations, fludarabine triphosphate inhibited human DNA ligase I activity directly by a mechanism which appeared to interfere with the formation of the adenosine monophosphate as a cofactor for the enzyme. In contrast, cytarabine triphosphate was inhibitory only at concentrations in excess of 1 mM which are generally not achieved during therapy [48]. Neither gemcitabine nor cladribine has been investigated for their effects on DNA ligation.

Self-Potentiation

The mechanism(s) by which the metabolites of a drug enhance the cytotoxicity of that drug is termed self-potentiation. This is most commonly brought about by the actions which either increase the accumulation of an active metabolite or which decrease its inactivation or elimination. As indicated by this name, it is expected that such actions would enhance the overall effects of the drug. No such activities have been identified for cytarabine. On the other hand, the ability of nucleotides of all three of the newer nucleoside antimetabolites to inhibit ribonucleotide reductase comprises a strong case for self-potentiation. Inhibition of ribonucleotide reductase is important because the activity of deoxycytidine kinase is regulated by deoxynucleotides such as dCTP and the phosphorylation of all the analogues is competitive with deoxycytidine. Because the cellular concentration of dCTP, and presumably deoxycytidine, is inversely proportional to kinase activity, inhibition of ribonucleotide reductase with the corresponding decrease in deoxynucleotides should increase the ability of a cell to phosphorylate the nucleotide antimetabolites. In addition, the natural deoxynucleotide triphosphates compete with the nucleotide analogues for incorporation into DNA. Lower cellular concentrations of the natural substrates would facilitate greater incorporation of the analogues into DNA, an action that is strongly correlated with cytotoxicity. Each of these actions, increased drug phosphorylation and a greater extent of incorporation into DNA, are likely to enhance the cytotoxicity of the drugs.

Gemcitabine has additional self-potentiation actions [40]. At high cellular concentrations, it appears that gemcitabine triphosphate inhibits the activity of CTP synthetase, the enzyme which converts UTP to CTP. By mass action, this may also have and effect on cellular dCTP levels. Gemcitabine monophosphate is known to be substrate for dCMP deaminase, which converts it to the corresponding uridine monophosphate analogue; this reaction essentially inactivates the drug. dCMP deaminase, however, requires dCTP as a cofactor, and when dCTP cellular levels are lowered, as is the case with gemcitabine inhibition of ribonucleotide reductase, gemcitabine monophosphate is not deaminated and remains as a substrate for phosphorylation to the active di- and triphosphates. Furthermore, gemcitabine triphosphate appears to compete with dCTP for activation of dCMP deaminase, and, at high cellular concentrations, may exert a second inhibitory effect on the activity of the enzyme. In summary, gemcitabine diphosphate inhibits the formation of deoxycytidine and its nucleotides by ribonucleotide reductase, and gemcitabine triphosphate may also affect the level of cellular cytidine nucleotides. Because there would be less deoxycytidine to compete for deoxycytidine kinase activity and possibly also for release of feedback inhibition of the enzyme, more gemcitabine should be phosphorylated and accumulate as the di- and triphosphates. The ratio of the cellular concentrations of gemcitabine triphosphate to dCTP would rise, facilitating additional incorporation of gemcitabine triphosphate into DNA with an increased cell kill. Lowering cellular dCTP levels would also reduce the inactivation of gemcitabine nucleotides by dCMP deaminase, and the activity of the enzyme would be further diminished at higher gemcitabine triphosphate concentrations. This should decrease the rate of gemcitabine triphosphate elimination, thus permitting prolongation of the inhibitory actions of the drug. Finally, the long residence time of gemcitabine nucleotides is likely to maintain inhibitory concentrations of the triphosphate for times sufficient to permit cycling cells to continue in the cell cycle until they enter the sensitive S phase to be killed.

Future Directions

Until recently, cytarabine was the drug of choice as an inhibitor of DNA repair in the design of therapeutic regimens. In general, the clinical results of such attempts at treating solid tumours have been disappointing. As detailed above, the newer nucleoside antimetabolites exhibit properties which should make them more effective inhibitors than cytarabine of both DNA replication and repair. Experimental evidence already exists for the synergistic interactions of fludarabine and radiation [49]. Other initiatives with gemcitabine and radiation are under way. Combinations of the nucleoside analogues and chemotherapeutic agents which elicit a DNA repair response are being explored. Studies which combined fludarabine with mitoxantrone [50], cisplatin and doxorubicin have already been translated into ongoing clinical trials. A phase I trial of chlorambucil and cladribine has recently been reported [26]. On a different tack, the potential of these new nucleosides to biochemically modulate the metabolism and activities of other drugs has also been exploited. The ability of fludarabine to activate the phosphorylation of cytarabine and to effectively double the concentration of cytarabine triphosphate has been demonstrated during clinical trials, and preliminary evaluations of phase II studies have demonstrated responses which are superior to cytarabine treatments without fludarabine [51,52]. We are only now recognising the potential of these new antimetabolites as single agents and as modulators of the metabolism and activities of other established drugs and modalities. Although it will be a major challenge to identify optimal doses, schedules and combinations, the present state of our knowledge of the pharmacokinetics, metabolism and actions of this class of antimetabolites promises that therapeutic rewards will be forthcoming in the future.

REFERENCES

1   Keating MJ, McCredie KB, Bodey GP, Smith TL, Gehan E, Freireich EJ: Unproved prospects for long term survival in adults with acute myelogenous leukemia. J Am Med Assoc 1982 (248):2481-2486

2   Velasquez W, Cabanillas F, Salvador P, McLaughlin P, Fridirk M, Tucker S, Jaganath S, Hagemeister FB, Redman JR, Swan F: Effective salvage therapy for lymphoma with cisplatin in combination with high-dose ara-C and dexamethasone (DHAP). Blood 1988 (71):117-122

3   Hertel LW, Boder GB, Kroin JS, Rinzel SM, Poore GA, Todd GC, Grindey GB: Evaluation of the antitumor activity of gemcitabine (2',2'-difluoro-2'-deoxycytidine). Cancer Res 1990 (50):4417-4422

4   LePage GA, Khaliq A, Gottleib JA: Studies of 9-ß-D-arabinofuranosyladenine in man. Drug Metab Dispo 1973 (1):756-759

5   Montgomery JA, Hewson K: An improved procedure for the preparation of 9-ß-D-arabinofuranosyl-2-fluoroadenine. J Heterocyc Chem 1979 (16):157-160

6   Simon LN, Bauer RJ, Tolman RL, Robins RK: Calf intestine adenosine deaminase. Substrate specificity. Biochemistry 1970 (9):573-577

7   Plunkett W, Gandhi V: Pharmacokinetics of arabinosylcytosine. J Infus Chemother 1992 (2):169-176

8   Liliemark JO, Plunkett W, Dixon DO: Relationship of 1-ß-D-arabinofuranosylcytosine in plasma to 1-ß-D-arabinofuranosylcytosine 5'-triphosphate level in leukemic cells during treatment with high-dose 1-ß-D-arabinofuranosylcytosine. Cancer Res 1985 (45): 5952-5957

9   Plunkett W, Liliemark JO, Adams TM, Nowak B, Estey E, Kantarjian H, Keating MJ: Saturation of 1-ß-D-arabinofuranosylcytosine 5'-triphosphate accumulation in leukemia cells during high-dose 1-ß-D-arabinofuranosylcytosine therapy. Cancer Res 1997 (47):3005-3011

10 Estey EH, Plunkett W, Kantarjian H, Rios MB, Keating MJ: Treatment of relapsed or refractory AML with intermediate-dose arabinosylcytosine (ara-C): confirmation of the importance of ara-C triphosphate formation in mediating response to ara-C. Leuk Lymph 1993 (10 Suppl):115-121

11 Heinemann V, Estey E, Keating MJ, Plunkett W: Patient-specific dose rate for continuous infusion high-dose arabinosylcytosine in relapsed acute myelogenous leukemia. J Clin Oncol 1989 (7):622-628

12 Ho DHW, Frei E III: Clinical Pharmacology of 1-ß-D-arabinofuranosyl cytosine. Clin Pharm Ther 1971 (12):944-954

13 Capizzi RL, Yang J-L, Cheng E, Bjornsson T, Sahasrabudhe D, Tan R-S, Cheng Y-C: Alteration of the pharmacokinetics of high-dose ara-C by its metabolite high ara-U in patients with acute leukemia. J Clin Oncol 1983 (1):763-771

14 Abbruzzese JL, Grunewald R, Weeks EA, Gravel D, Adams T, Nowak B, Mineishi S, Tarassoff P, Satterlee W, Raber MN, Plunkett W: A phase I clinical, plasma, and cellular pharmacology study of gemcitabine. J Clin Oncol 1991 (9):491-498

15 Grunewald R, Kantarjian H, Du M, Faucher K, Tarassoff P, Plunkett W: Gemcitabine in leukemia: a phase I clinical, plasma, and cellular pharmacology study. J Clin Oncol 1992 (10):406-413

16 Plunkett W, Gandhi V, Chubb S, Nowak B, Heinemann V, Mineishi S, Sen A, Hertel LW, Grindey GB: 2',2'-difluorodeoxycytidine metabolism and mechanism of action in human leukemia cells. Nucleoside Nucleotide 1989 (8):775-785

17 Grunewald R, Abbruzzese JL, Tarassoff P, Plunkett W: Saturation of 2',2'-difluorodeoxycytidine 5'-triphosphate accumulation by mononuclear cells during a phase I trial of gemcitabine. Cancer Chemother Pharm 1991 (27):258-262

18 Grunewald R, Kantarjian H, Keating MJ, Abbruzzese JL, Tarassoff P, Plunkett W: Pharmacologically directed design of the dose rate and schedule of 2',2'-difluorodeoxycytidine (Gemcitabine) administration in leukemia. Cancer Res 1990 (50):6823-6826

19 Keating MJ, O'Brien S, Kantarjian H, Plunkett W, Estey E, Koller C, Beran M, Freireich EJ: Long-term follow-up of patients with chronic lymphocytic leukemia treated with fludarabine as a single agent. Blood 1993 (81):2878-2884

20 Hersh M, Kuhn JG, Philips JL, Clark G, Ludden TM, Von Hoff DD: Pharmacokinetic study of fludarabine monophosphate (NSC 312887). Cancer Chemother Pharm 1986 (17):277-280

21 Danhauser L, Plunkett W, Keating MJ, Cabanillas F: 9-ß-D-arabinofuranosyl-2-fluoroadenine 5'-monophosphate pharmacokinetics in plasma and tumor cells of patients with relapsed leukemia and lymphoma. Cancer Chemother Pharmacol 1986 (18):145-152

22 Malspeis L, Grever MR, Staubus AE, Young D: Pharmacokinetics of 2-F-ara-A (9-ß-D-arabinofuranosyl-2-fluoroadenine) in cancer patients during the phase I clinical investigations of fludarabine phosphate. Sem Oncol 1990 (17 Suppl):18-32

23 Kemena A, Fernandez M, Bauman J, Keating MJ, Plunkett W: A sensitive fluorescence assay for quantitation of fludarabine and metabolites in biological fluids. Clin Chim Acta 1991 (200):95-106

24 Avramis VI, Champagne J, Sato J, Krailo M, Ettinger LJ, Poplack DG, Finkelstein J, Reaman G, Hammond GD, Holcenberg JS: Pharmacology of fludarabine phosphate after a phase I/II trial by a loading bolus and continuous infusion in pediatric patients. Cancer Res 1990 (50):7226-7231

25 Liliemark JO, Juliusson G: On the pharmacokinetics of 2-chlorodeoxyadenosine in humans. Cancer Res 1991 (51):5570-5572

26 Tefferia A, Witzig TE, Reid JM, Li C-Y, Ames MM: Phase I study of combined 2-chlorodeoxyadenosine and chlorambucil in chronic lymphoid leukemia and low-grade lymphoma. J Clin Oncol 1994 (12):569-574

27 Kessel D: Some observations of the phosphorylation of cytosine arabinoside. Mol Pharmacol 1968 (4):402-404

28 Heinemann V, Hertel LW, Grindey GB, Plunkett W: Comparison of the cellular pharmacokinetics and toxicity of 2',2'-difluorodeoxycytidine and 1-ß-D-

arabinofuranosylcytosine. Cancer Res 1988 (48):4024-4031

29 Krenitsky TA, Tuttle JV, Koszalka GW, Chen IS, Beacham LM III, Rideout JL, Elion GB: Deoxycytidine kinase from calf thymus. Substrate and inhibitor specificity. J Biol Chem 1976 (252):4055-4061

30 Bennett LL Jr, Chang C-H, Allan PW, Adamson JJ, Fose LM, Brockman RW, Secrist JA III, Shortnacy A, Montgomery JA: Metabolism and metabolic effects of halopurine nucleosides in tumor cells in culture. Nucleosides Nucleotides 1985 (4):107-116

31 Avrey TL, Rehg JE, Lumm WCC, Harwood FC, Santana V, Blakley RL: Biochemical pharmacology of 2-chlorodeoxyadenosine in malignant human hematopoietic cell lines and therapeutic effects of 2-bromodeoxyadenosine in drug combinations in mice. Cancer Res 1989 (49):4972-4978

32 Shewach DS, Reynolds KK, Hertel L: Nucleotide specificity of human deoxycytidine kinase. Mol. Pharmacol. 1992 (42):518-524

33 Kemena A, Gandhi V, Shewach DS, Keating M, Plunkett W: Inhibition of fludarabine metabolism by arabinosylcytosine during therapy. Cancer Chemother Pharm 1992 (31):193-199

34 White EL, Shaddix SC, Brockman RW, Bennett LL Jr: Comparison of the action of 9-ß-D-arabinofuranosyl-2-fluoroadenine and 9-ß-D-arabinofuranosyladenine on target enzymes from mouse tumor cells. Cancer Res 1982 (42):2260-2264

35 Parker WB, Bapat AR, Shen J-X, Townsend AJ, Cheng Y-C: Interaction of 2-halogenated dATP analogs (F, Cl, Br) with human DNA polymerases, DNA primase and ribonucleotide reductase. Mol Pharmacol 1988 (34):485-491

36 Heinemann V, Xu Y-Z, Chubb S, Sen A, Hertel LW, Grindey GB, Plunkett W: Inhibition of ribonucleotide reduction in CCRF-CEM cells by 2',2'-difluorodeoxycytidine. Mol Pharmacol 1990 (38):567-572

37 Baker CH, Banzon J Bollinger JM, Stubbe J, Samano V, Robins MJ, Lippert B, Jarvi E, Resvick R: 2'-Deoxy-2'-methylenecytidine and 2'-deoxy-2',2'-difluorodeoxycytidine 5'-diphosphates: potent mechanism-based inhibitors of ribonucleotide reductase. J Med Chem 1991 (34):1879-1884

38 Moore EC and Cohen SS: Effects of arabinosylnucleotides on ribonucleotide reduction by an enzyme system form rat tumor. J Biol Chem 1967 (242):2116-2118

39 Plunkett W and Gandhi V: Cellular pharmacodynamics of anticancer drugs. Sem Oncol 1993 (20):50-63

40 Heinemann V, Xu Y-Z, Chubb S, Sen A, Hertel LW, Grindey GB, Plunkett W: Cellular elimination of 2',2' difluorodeoxycytidine 5'-triphosphate: a mechanism of self-potentiation. Cancer Res 1992 (52):533-539

41 Major PP, Egan EM, Herrick DJ, Kufe DW: Effect of ara-C incorporation on deoxyribonucleic acid synthesis in cells. Biochem Pharm 1982 (31):2937-2940

42 Hentosh P, Koob R, Blakley RL: Incorporation of 2-halogeno-2'-deoxyadenosine 5-triphosphates into DNA during replication by human polymerases a and b. J Biol Chem 1990 (265):4033-4040

43 Huang P, Chubb S, Plunkett W: Termination of DNA synthesis by 9-ß-D-arabinofuranosyl-2-fluoroadenine. A mechanism for cytotoxicity. J Biol Chem 1990 (265):16617-16625

44 Huang P, Chubb S, Hertel LW, Grindey GB, Plunkett W: Action of 2',2'-difluorodeoxycytidine on DNA synthesis. Cancer Res 1991 (51):6110-6117

45 Kamiya K, Huang P, Plunkett W: Mechanism of inhibition of the 3'->5' exonuclease activity of human DNA polymerase epsilon by DNA containing fludarabine nucleotide. Proc. Am Assn Cancer Res 1994 (35):393

46 Mikita T, Beardsley GP: Functional consequences of the arabinosylcytosine structural lesion in DNA. Biochemistry 1988 (27):4698-4705

47 Yang S-W, Huang P, Plunkett W, Becker FF, Chan JYH: Dual mode of inhibition of purified DNA ligase I from human cells by 9-ß-D-arabinofuranosyl-2-fluoroadenine triphosphate. J Biol Chem 1992 (267): 2345-2349

48 Zittoun J, Marquet J, David JC: Mechanism of inhibition of DNA ligase in ara-C treated cells. Leukemia Res 1991 (15):157-164

49 Gregoire V, Hunter N, Milas L, Brock WA, Plunkett W, Hittelman W: Potentiation of radiation-induced regrowth delay in murine tumors by fludarabine. Cancer Res 1994 (54):468-474

50 McLaughlin P, Hagemeister FB, Swan F, Cabanillas F, Pate O, Romaguera JE, Rodriguez MA, Redman JR, Keating MJ: Phase I study of the combination fludarabine, mitoxantrone, and dexamethasone in low-grade lymphoma. J Clin Oncol 1994 (12):575-579

51 Estey E, Plunkett W, Gandhi V, Rios MB, Kantarjian H, Keating MJ: Fludarabine and arabinosylcytosine therapy of refractory and relapsed acute myelogenous leukemia. Leukemia Lymphoma 1993 (9):343-350

52 Gandhi V, Estey E, Keating MJ, Plunkett W: Fludarabine potentiates metabolism of cytarabine in patients with acute myelogenous leukemia during therapy. J Clin Oncol 1993 (11):116-124

Thymidylate Synthase Inhibitors, Modulation of 5-Fluorouracil and Folate Analogues

Peter Harper [1] and Hilary Calvert [2]

1 Department of Medical Oncology, Guy's Hospital, St. Thomas Street, London SE1 9RT, United Kingdom
2 Division of Oncology, Newcastle General Hospital, Newcastle upon Tyne NE4 6BE, United Kingdom

The fluorinated pyrimidines were first reported as a class of tumour inhibitory compounds more than 30 years ago and 5-fluorouracil rapidly entered into clinical practice. The effects of 5-fluorouracil on the cell are 1) inhibition of thymidylate synthase, 2) a direct effect on DNA, and 3) a direct effect on RNA [1]. These mechanisms and their modulation by other factors designed to increase activation, response rates and survival, will be discussed in this chapter.

The Effect of 5-FU on Thymidylate Synthase

The initial evidence was that the antitumour effect of 5-fluorouracil (5-FU) was mediated through the inhibition of thymidylate synthase (TS). The metabolism of 5-FU led to the production of 5-fluorodeoxyuridine monophosphate (FdUMP) to substitute and compete for the naturally occurring uridine-monophosphate (UMP). The FdUMP inhibits the action of thymidylate synthase, decreasing the production of deoxythymidine monophosphate and thus preventing the formation of thymidylate, the essential precursor of deoxythymidine triphosphate (DTTP), one of 4 deoxyribonucleotides required for DNA synthesis. To enable a satisfactory degree and duration of inhibition of thymidylate synthase, a ternary complex has to be produced consisting of thymidylate synthase, FdUMP and a co-factor consisting of 5, 10, methyline-tetrahydrofolate. The production of the nucleotide fluoruridine triphosphate (FUTP) impairs RNA processing and function.

Figure 1 sets out in outline the metabolic pathways of 5-fluorouracil.

Direct Effect on DNA

Fluorouracil by direct effect on DNA results in strand breakage, perhaps resulting in incomplete DNA repair consequent to deoxyribonucleotide depletion or from attempts to excise and repair DNA containing 5FU.

Direct Effect on RNA

Incorporation of 5-FU into RNA may result from irreversible inhibition of RNA methylation affecting protein synthesis.

Modulation of 5-Fluorouracil

Modulation of the activity of fluorouracil is intended to enhance activation and increase the therapeutic window of tumour inhibition. These mechanisms have recently been reviewed by Kobayashi and Schilsky [2] and were also discussed in the excellent overall review of the fluorinated pyrimidines by Jean Grem [3].
The most commonly exploited modulation of fluorouracil is alteration in the availability of reduced folates to affect the ternary complex (TS, FdUMP, reduced folate) [4]. Calcium folinate (calcium leucovorin) is itself a recemic mixture of two stereoisomers D and L. The L

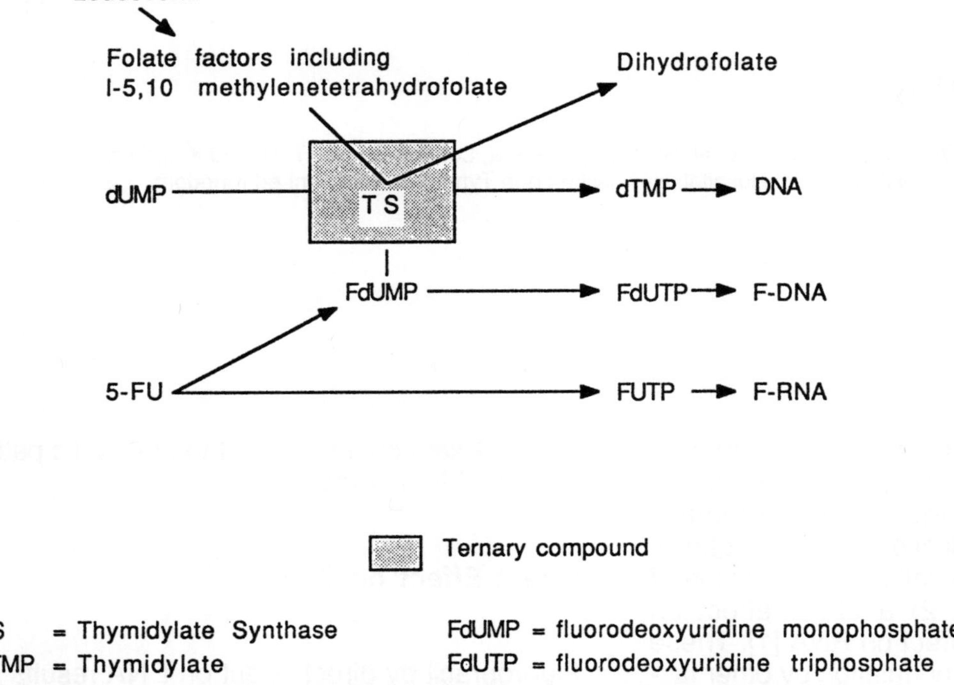

Fig. 1. Metabolic pathway of fluoropyrimidines and the effect of folate precursors

isomer alone is the pharmacologically active one and it is now becoming available commercially. The folate co-factors are themselves metabolised to polyglutamate derivatives [5]. The intracellular retention of these cofactors depends in part on the length of the polyglutamate chain and the binding of the cofactors to TS is also greater with longer chain lengths [5]. It is therefore both the absolute level of polyglutamate pool and the polyglutamate chain length which will determine the degree and duration of inhibition of TS. Dose of leucovorin administered, schedule of administration (for instance i.v. push, short-term infusion or long-term infusion), oral or intravenous administration will all affect this outcome. These underlying effects must be taken into account in the design of clinical studies and in the interpretation of those studies. It is clear that one method and one dose may not necessarily be the same as another schedule and great care must be taken in the comparison of clinical trials.

In the meta-analysis of advanced colorectal cancer trials, reported to the Journal of Clinical Oncology, single-agent 5-FU has an overall response rate of 11% and 5-FU leucovorin-primed schedules had an overall reponse rate

of 23% [6]. The optimal dose of fluorouracil and leucovorin have not been determined though for many clinicians the results of the large randomised trial of the Gastrointestinal Study Group (GITSG) [7] or the North Central Cancer Treatment Group set out reasonable schedules [8,9].

Petrelli in 1989 reported on behalf of the Gastrointestinal Study Group with a comparison of 3 regimens: 5-fluorouracil used alone in a dose of 500 mg daily x 5 repeated on a 4-week basis, compared with 2 leucovorin-primed regimens used weekly for 6 out of each 8 weeks. The leucovorin priming was at 500 mg (high-dose folinic acid) or 25 mg (low-dose folinic acid) with the fluorouracil dose kept at 600 mg in each arm. There was a significant improvement in response rate for the high-dose leucovorin arm, some prolongation in the median duration of response but overall no alteration in survival. Toxicity showed no major changes in nausea and vomiting for any of the regimens, there was some increase in diarrhoea with the high-dose leucovorin regimen but no increase in mucositis.

Erlichman [10] reported on the Toronto study, which again showed an improvement in response rate for the leucovorin-primed 5-FU and an alteration in survival (54 weeks versus 51 weeks) just reaching statistical significance.

Other methods of modulation of 5-FU include increase in its activation, alteration of the nucleotide pool, and further enhancement of DNA or RNA-mediated activity. The mechanisms are varied.

The largest randomised study was that of the NCCTG [9] comparing 3 schedules, 5-FU alone, 500 mg/m2 i.v. push, 5-FU 370 mg/m2 push with leucovorin 200 mg/m2 i.v. push (HDFA), and 5-FU 370 mg/m2 push with leucovorin 20 mg/m2 i.v. push (LDFA). There was a significant survival advantage for both the leucovorin-treated arms over 5-FU alone (12 months vs 5 months) with the LDFA arm also being positive on quality of life parameters.

Increase in Activation of 5-FU

Further modulation of fluorouracil can take place with the alteration of the activity of 5-FU by its anabolic enzymes affecting the conversion to 5-FdUMP and 5-FUTP. Antifolates and purine synthesis inhibitors will also alter the availability of phosphoribosyl pyrophosphate (PRP) (vide infra).

Reduction of the Nucleotide Pool

The natural nucleotide pool (dUMP and UTP) can be reduced by the action of hydroxyurea and N-(phosphonoacetyl)-L-aspartate (PALA) which is an inhibitor of L-aspartate transcarbamylase. By reduction of dUMP and UTP pools there is less competition for 5FdUMP [3]. Kemeny et al. [11] giving Pala 24 hours prior to 5-FU obtained an objective tumour regression in 35% of patients with advanced colorectal cancer. O'Dwyer et al. achieved response rates of 43%. Toxicity includes the classic side-effects of fluorouracil alone (stomatitis, diarrhoea, bone marrow suppression and rash) with an increase in cerebellar ataxia and a syndrome of hyperbilirubinaemia, ascites and hypoalbuminaemia [12]. This latter syndrome proved largely reversible with discontinuation of therapy and was frequently observed in patients with tumour response.

Depletion of Folate Cofactors and Inhibition of Purine Synthesis

Methotrexate, by inhibition of dihydrofolate reductate, results in depletion of the intracellular pools of reduced folate cofactors and inhibition of purine synthesis. Phosphoribosyl pyrophosphate (PRPP), a phosphate group donor, is therefore more available to activate 5-fluorouracil to 5-UMP. Marsh et al. reported on this combination in the treatment of advanced colorectal cancer with methotrexate at 200 mg/m2 followed by 5-FU given either 1 or 24 hours later and found a significant improvement in response rate and survival in favour of the 24-hour interval [13,14].

5-Fluorouracil and alpha interferon have an apparent synergistic action, though the mechanism of the effect is not fully understood [2]. There appears to be enhanced conversion of 5-FU to 5-FdUMP, some inhibition of thymidine salvage pathways and inhibition of the rise in intracellular thymidylate synthase observed following exposure to 5-fluorouracil. Clinical trials have not as yet shown an improvement in response or survival [15-17].

Protracted Infusion of 5-FU

Continuous infusion of fluorouracil both alone and with modulation by leucovorin continues to demonstrate high response rates in advanced colorectal cancer, in which it has been extensively tested. These protracted infusional schedules are being used as a method of enhancing fluorouracil activity. Seifert reported in 1975 on a comparison of continuous infusion versus bolus fluorouracil and demonstrated response rates of 42% versus 20% [18]. Kish [14] reported in 1985 in head and neck cancer response rates of the continuous infusion arm of 72% versus 20% for the bolus arms. Lockich, reporting on the mid-Atlantic Oncology programme in colon cancer, demonstrated a response rate for continuous infusion FU (10 weeks duration) of 30% whereas for bolus 5-FU the response rate was 7% [20]. Leukopenia occurred in 38% of patients receiving bolus 5-FU and there was no significant leukopenia in those with infusion chemotherapy. Hand and foot syndrome were not seen at all in the bolus arm but occurred in 23% of those patients receiving infusional chemotherapy.

Conclusion

Overall, modulation of the effects of 5-FU are resulting in improvement in response rates; however, there is no consistent improvement in survival and there is clearly demonstrated alteration in toxicity. Lack of effects on survival overall are not surprising given this lack of consistency of the effect of treatment on survival. Trial size is on the whole small and there is considerable variation in the scheduling and dose of fluorouracil and its modulates which make a considerable difference to activity and response rates. There is considerable heterogeneity in the patient groups, however, within the few more recent and larger studies there have been significant improvements for subsets of patients both in disease-free interval and survival. Large, well conducted trials will be needed to demonstrate the consistency of these claims. Given the large number of patients with colorectal cancer presenting each year, even small increases in survival will result in a great many patients benefitting. Quality-of-life parameters should also be included in the results.

The design of more specific thymidylate synthase inhibitors has now been accomplished.

Folate-Based Thymidylate Synthase Inhibitors

As reported earlier, the evidence suggests that the antitumour effects of 5-fluorouracil are mediated through the inhibition of thymidylate synthase (TS) by 5-fluorodeoxyuridine monophosphate (FdUMP), a metabolite of 5-FU [2]. It has been argued that the inhibition of TS should be better achieved by a folate analogue [22]. 5-FU requires metabolic activation, a process that may be deficient in some cells, and subsequently has to compete with deoxyuridine monophosphate (dUMP) for binding to TS [1]. The feedback control of the pyrimidine *de novo* pathway means that dUMP levels increase dramatically following inhibition of TS and can compete with FdUMP for TS binding. The incorporation of 5-FU metabolites into DNA and RNA may have a role in generating the side-effects observed with 5-FU as may the generation of potentially toxic degradation products such as 2-fluoro-ß-alanine [21]. In contrast, a folate analogue does not require activation and the competing substrate, 5,10-methylenetetrahydrofolate, cannot accumulate since, being a vitamin, there is no synthetic pathway. Similarly, it cannot be incorporated into nucleic acids and is unlikely to be degraded [22]. These considertations led to the synthesis of folate analogues designed specifically to inhibit TS while not affecting other folate-dependent reactions such as dihydrofolate reductase. The first of these was CB 3717 [22] (Fig. 2).

Clinical Results with CB 3717

Phase I studies with CB 3717 demonstrated a number of toxicities (malaise, abnormal liver function tests, rashes) with nephrotoxicity as dose-limiting toxicity. Myelosuppression was sporadic and occasionally severe [23]. Several responses were observed and subsequent phase II trials showed activity in pre-treated breast and ovarian cancer patients, although there was no activity in mesothelioma or colon cancer (Table 1) [24,25,27]. Of the 8 responding patients with breast cancer, 3 were reported as resistant to prior therapy, 2 as responding to prior therapy and 3 had not received prior therapy.

These results indicated at least a degree of activity for this antimetabolite in heavily pre-treated patients with the two solid tumours, breast and ovarian cancer. However, CB 3717 did not progress into clinical development be-

Table 1. Phase II results with CB 3717

	Total patients	Partial response
Breast	52	8
Ovarian	45	8
Colon	25	0
Mesothelioma	18	1

cause of sporadic life-threatening toxicity. Of 173 patients in phase II studies 16 experienced toxicity consisting of renal failure, myelosuppression and gastrointestinal toxicity. Eight of these patients died [27]. A multivariate analysis failed to elucidate pretreatment characteristics to allow the patients at risk to be identified. For this reason the clinical development of CB 3717 was abandoned.

Second Generation Inhibitors

The Search for More Soluble Derivatives

The clinical responses observed with CB 3717 served as a catalyst for the development of alternative folate-based TS inhibitors with a more favourable therapeutic profile. Analogues have been pursued by several pharmaceutical companies as well as by academic groups. The first priority was clearly to identify the cause of the sporadic but serious toxicity so that it could be "designed out" of an analogue. The clinical pattern of toxicities suggested that the renal failure was the precipitating event, followed by drug retention and the subsequent development of gut and bone marrow toxicity due to the antiproliferative effects of the drug. It was shown that the solubility of CB 3717, although reasonable at neutral pH, diminished drastically as the pH reduced and was minimal at pH 4-5, the normal pH of urine. When acidified CB 3717 solutions tended to form a gel rather than precipitate. This suggested that the nephrotoxicity of CB 3717 was due to obstruction of the renal tubules. Trials of CB 3717 with alkalinization failed to resolve the problem [28]. Jones et al. [29] speculated that the insolubility of CB 3717 was due to intermolecular hydrogen bonding involving the 2-amino substituent and therefore synthesised the 2-desamino analogue. This displayed markedly greater aqueous solubility and, surprisingly, only reduced the inhibitory potency towards TS by about 10-fold. Subsequently it was found that substitution of a methyl group at the 2 position restored most of the inhibitory potency associated with CB 3717, but also preserved the enhanced solubility of the desamino analogue [30].

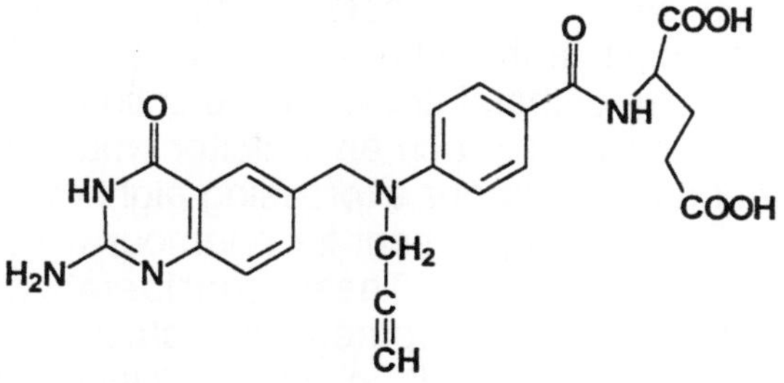

CB 3717

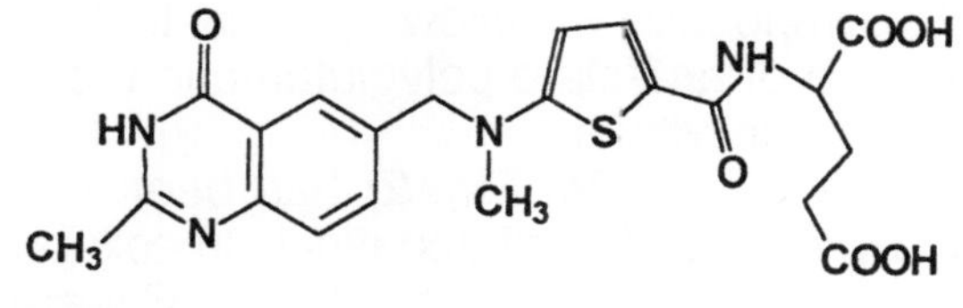

ZD 1694

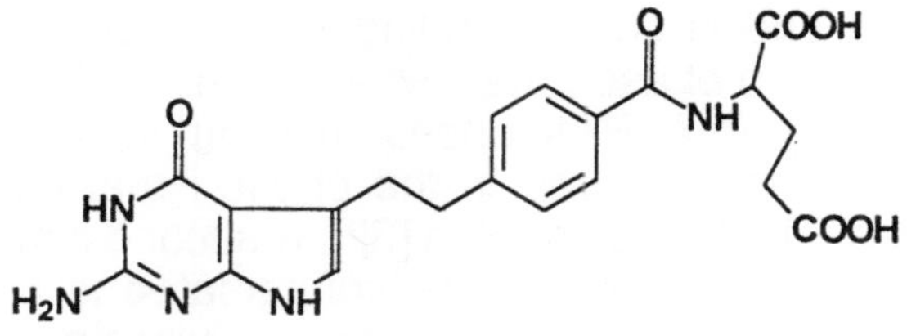

LY 231514

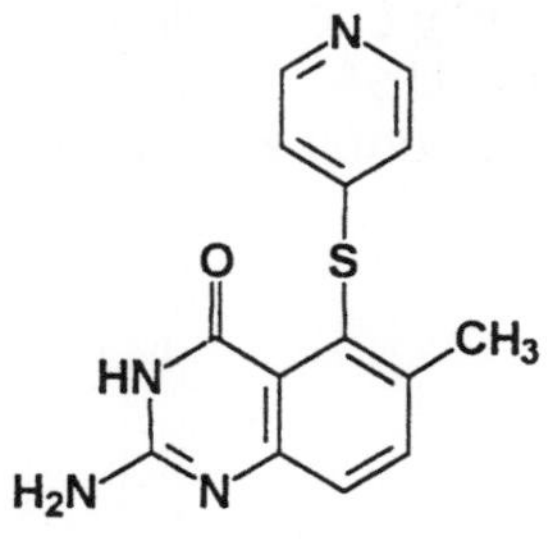

AG 337

Fig. 2. Folate-based thymidylate synthase inhibitors which have been or are in clinical trials

The Role of Polyglutamation

Polyglutamates of naturally occurring folates are retained within the cell and may be better substrates for the enzymes involved in folate metabolism. Many folate analogues are also substrates for the enzyme, folylpolyglutamate synthetase (FPGS). In the case of many thymidylate synthase inhibitors, the polyglutamate derivatives are substantially more effective as inhibitors than their monoglutamate counterparts [31]. A TS inhibitor that is readily converted to polyglutamates will be more potent both because the polyglutamate derivatives possess enhanced activity against TS and because of their intracellular retention. The therapeutic ratio of such an inhibitor would be enhanced for a tumour expressing high levels of FPGS but low or absent for a tumour which expressed low levels. These considerations have led to the development of 2 classes of analogues. Compounds in the first class are avid substrates for FPGS while those in the second are non-substrates. The current trials of these compounds will allow a clinical test of the relevance of antifolate polyglutamation to antitumour selectivity.

Tomudex (ZD 1694, Fig. 2) has been developed by Zeneca Pharmaceuticals in collaboration with the Institute of Cancer Research (England). This drug is an avid substrate for FPGS and is correspondingly potent both *in vitro* and in phase I trials where it has an MTD of 3.5 mg/m². Responses of solid tumours have been observed in the phase I trial and phase II trials are ongoing [32]. A second compound which is readily polyglutamated is LY 231514. Preclinically this shows activity similar to that of tomudex but with reduced weight loss in animals [33]. It is currently undergoing phase I studies in the UK and the USA.

The development of compounds which are not substrates for FPGS has resulted in both "classic", relatively hydrophilic, analogues and lipophilic inhibitors. The d-dimensional structure of TS (first published by Stroud et al. in 1987 [24]) has allowed the development of "designer" TS inhibitors which would not have been possible using the classic techniques of medicinal chemistry. Two compounds which have been developed by the Agouron Pharmaceutical Company (AG 331 and Ag 337, Fig. 2) are currently in phase I clinical trials [25].

Summary and Conclusions

The majority of indications for antimetabolites have always been in the treatment of leukaemias and this class of compounds has been perceived as having only a minimal role in the treatment of solid tumours. Nevertheless, current evidence suggests that the target of TS may have a significant role in the treatment of solid tumours, particularly colorectal cancer, a group where adjuvant therapy with 5-fluorouracil has been shown to improve survival. Studies with the newer folate-based inhibitors of the same target also suggest that attack of this locus will result in solid tumour activity.

REFERENCES

1 Pinedo HM, Peter GFJ: Fluorouracil: biochemistry and pharmacology. J Clin Oncol 1988 (6):1653-1664
2 Kobayashi K, Schilsky R: Update on biochemical modulation of chemotherapeutic agents. Oncology 1993 (7):99-109
3 Grem JL: Fluoropyrimidines. In Chabner BA and Collins JM (eds) Pharmacologic Principles of Cancer Treatment, 2nd Ed. J. Saunders, Philadelphia 1990 pp 180-224
4 Santi DV, McHenry CS, Sommer H: Mechanism of interaction of thymidylate synthetase with 5-fluoro-deoxyuridylate. Biochemistry 1974 (13):471-481
5 Radparvar S, Houghton PJ, Houghton JA: Effect of polyglutamylation of 5,10-methylenetetrahydrofolate on the binding of 5-fluoro-2'-deoxyuridylate to thymidylate synthase purified from a human colon adenocarcinoma xenograft. Biochem Pharmacol 1989 (38):335-342
6 Advanced Colorectal Cancer Metaanalysis Project: Modulation of fluorouracil by leucovorin in patients with advanced colorectal cancer. J Clin Oncol 1992 (10):896-903
7 Petrelli N, Douglass HO Jr, Herrera L et al: The modulation of fluorouracil with leucovorin in metastatic colorectal carcinoma. J Clin Oncol 1989 (7): 1419-1426
8 Poon MA, O'Connell MJ, Moertel CG et al: Biochemical modulation of fluorouracil: evidence of significant improvement of survival and quality of life in patients with advanced colorectal carcinoma. J Clin Oncol 1989 (7):1407-1418
9 O'Connell MJ: A controlled clinical trial including folinic acid at two distinct dose levels in combination with 5-fluorouracil (5FU) for the treatment of advanced colorectal cancer; experience of the Mayo Clinical and North Central Cancer Treatment Group. In: Ruthum Y and McGuire JJ (eds) The Expanding Role of Folates and Fluoropyrimidines in Cancer Chemotherapy: Advances in Experimental Medicine and Biology. Plenum Press, New York 1988 pp 173-182
10 Erlichman C, Fine S, Wong A et al: A randomized trial of fluorouracil and folinic acid in patients with metastatic colorectal carcinoma. J Clin Oncol 1988 (6):469-475
11 Kemeny N, Conti JA, Seiter K et al: Biochemical modulation of bolus fluorouracil by PALA in patients with advanced colorecal cancer. J Clin Oncol 1992 (10):747-752
12 Kemeny N, Seiter K, Urmacher C et al: A new syndrome: Ascites, hyperbilirubinemia, and hypoalbuminemia in association with bichemical modulation of fluorouracil. Am Intern Med 1991 (115):946-951
13 Marsh JC, Bertino JR, Katz KH et al: The influence of drug interval on the effect of methotrexate and fluorouracil in the treatment of advanced colorectal cancer. J Clin Oncol 1991 (9):371-380
14 Kemeny N, Ahmed T, Michaelson R et al: Activity of sequential low-dose methotrexate and fluorouracil in advanced colorectal carcinoma: An attempt at correlation with tissue and blood levels of phosphoribosylpyrophosphate. J Clin Oncol 1984 (2):311-315
15 Kemeny N, Younes A, Seiter K et al: Interferon alpha-2a and 5-fluorouracil for advanced colorectal carcinoma. Assessment of activity and toxicity. Cancer 1990 (66):2470-2475
16 Pazdur R, Ajani JA, Patt YZ et al: Phase II study of fluorouracil and recombinant interferon alfa-2a in previously untreated advanced colorectal carcinoma. J Clin Oncol 1990 (8):2027-2031
17 Wadler S, Lembersky B, Atkins M et al: Phase II trial of fluorouracil and recombinant interferon alfa-2a in patients with advanced colorecal carcinoma: An Eastern Cooperative Oncology Group Study. J Clin Oncol 1991 (9):1806-1810
18 Seifert P, Baker LH, Reed ML et al: Comparison of continuously infused 5-fluorouracil with bolus injection in treatment of patients with colorectal adenocarcinoma. Cancer 1975 (36):123-128
19 Kish JA, Ensley JF, Jacobs J et al: A randomized trial of cisplatin and 5-fluorouracil (5FU) and cisplatin and 5FU bolus for recurrent and advanced squamous cell carcinoma of the head and neck. Cancer 1985 (56):2740-2744
20 Lokich J, Ahlgren J, Gullo J et al: A prospective randomized comparison of continuous infusion fluorouracil with a conventional bolus schedule in metastatic colorectal carcinoma: a mid-Atlantic Oncology Programme Study. J Clin Oncol 1989 (7): 425-432
21 Jackman AL, Jones TR, Calvert AH: Thymidylate synthetase inhibitors: experimental and clinical aspects. In: Muggia FM (ed) Experimental and Clinical Progress in Cancer Chemotherapy. Martinus Nijhoff, Boston 1985 pp 155-210
22 Jones TR, Calvert AH, Jackman AL, Brown SJ, Jones M, Harrap KR: A potent antitumour quinazoline inhibitor of thymidylate synthetase: synthesis, biological properties and therapeutic results in mice. Eur J Cancer 1981 (17):11-19
23 Calvert AH, Alison DL, Harland SJ, Jackman AL, Jones TR, Newell DR, Siddik ZH, Wiltshaw E, McElwain TJ, Smith IE and Harrap KR: A phase I evaluation of the quinazoline antifolate thymidylate synthetase inhibitor N10-propargyl-5, 8-dideazafolic acid. J Clin Oncol 1986 (4/8):1245-1252
24 Cantwell BMJ, Macaulay V, Harris AL, Kaye SB, Smith IE, Milstead RAV, Calvert AH: Phase II study of the antifolate N10-propargyl-5, 8 dideazafolic acid (CB3717) in advanced breast cancer. Eur J Cancer Clin Oncol 1988 (24):733-736
25 Harding MJ, Cantwell BM, Milstead RA, Harris AL, Kaye SB: Phase II study of the thymidylate synthetase inhibitor CB3717 (N10-propargyl-5, 8-dideazafolic acid) in colorectal cancer. Br J Cancer 1988 (57):628-629
26 Cantwell BM, Earnshaw M, Harris AL: Phase II study of a novel antifolate, N10-propargyl-5,8 dideazafolic acid (CB3717) in malignant mesothelioma. Cancer Treat Rep 1986 (70):1335-1336
27 Harrap KR, Jackman AL, Newell DR, Taylor GA, Hughes LR, Calvert AH: Thymidylate synthase: A target for anticancer drug design. Advances in Enzyme Regulation 1989 (29):161-179

28 Calvert AH, Newell DR, Jackman AL, Gumbrell LA, Sikora E, Grzelakowska-Sztabert B, Bishop J, Judson IR, Harland SJ, Harrap KR: Recent preclinical and clinical studies with the thymidylate synthase inhibitor N10-propargyl-5, 8-dideazafolic acid (CB3717). NCI Monograph 1987 (5):231-218

29 Jones TR, Thornton TJ, Flinn A, Jackman AL, Newell DR, Calvert AH: Quinazoline antifolates inhibiting thymidylate synthase: 2-desamino derivatives with enhanced solubility and potency. J Med Chem 1989 (32 /4):847-852

30 Hughes LR, Jackman AL, Oldfield J, Smith RC, Burrows KD, Marsham PR, Bishop JA, Jones TR, O'Connor BM, Calvert AH: Quinazoline antifolate thymidylate synthase inhibitors: alkyl, substituted alkyl, and aryl substituents in the C2 position. J Med Chem 1990 (33/11):3060-3067

31 Sikora E, Jackman AL, Newell DR, Calvert AH: Formation and retention and biological activity of N10-propargyl-5, 8-dideazafolic acid (CB3717) polyglutamates in L1210 cells in vitro. Biochem Pharmacol 1988 (37):4047-4054

32 Judson I, Clarke S, Ward J, Planting A, Verweij J, de Boer M, Spiers J, Smith R, Sutcliffe F: A phase I trial of the thymidylate synthase inhibitor, ICI D1694. Ann Oncol 1993 (3 suppl 5):51 (abstract)

33 Grindey GB, Shih C, Barnett CJ, Pearce HL, Englehardt JA, Todd GC, Rinzel SM, Worzalla JF, Gosset LS, Everson TP, Wilson TM, Kobierski ME, Winter MA, Bewley JR, Kuhnt D, Taylor EC, Moran RG: Ly231514, a novel pyrrolopyrimidine antifolate that inhibits thymidylate synthase (TS). Proc Am Assoc Cancer Res 1992 (33):411

34 Hardy LW, Finer-Moore JS, Montfort WR, Jones MO, Santi DV, Stroud RM: Atomic structure of thymidylate synthase: target for rational drug design. Science 1987 (235):448-455

35 Taylor GA, Rafi I, Balmanno K, Calvete JA, Newell DR, Webber S, Jackson RC, Gumbrell L, Chapman F, Oakey A, Proctor M, Simmons D, Lind MJ, Bailey N, Calvert AH: Preclinical and early clinical studies with the lipophilic thymidylate synthase inhibitor, AG 337. Br J Cancer 1994 (67 suppl XX):17

A Review of Fludarabine and Cladribine in Solid Tumours

Gilbert B. Zulian

Department of Onco-Haematology, Geneva University Hospital, 1211 Geneva 14, Switzerland

Fludarabine monophosphate (FAMP) and cladribine (CDA) are adenosine analogues that were shown to be highly active in the management of lymphoid malignancies such as hairy cell leukaemia, low-grade non-Hodgkin's lymphoma, chronic lymphocytic leukaemia, Waldenström macroglobulinaemia and cutaneous T-cell lymphoma [1,2]. Both have also been used in acute leukaemias and fludarabine appears particularly promising for this indication [3]. Activation of FAMP and CDA is realised through phosphorylation by deoxycytidine kinase (dCTk) to their respective triphosphate compounds and both are degraded by 5'-nucleotidase (5'-NT). As opposed to their physiologic counterparts, FAMP and CDA are resistant to deamination by adenosine deaminase (ADA). The balance between activation and degradation appears crucial for their clinical activity [4]. FAMP and CDA are cytotoxic not by inducing necrosis but rather programmed cell death, apoptosis, by means of activation of specific endonucleases [5].

In solid tumours, however, the situation is quite different as no clinical activity has been demonstrated so far for either agent. The available data are presented in this paper for both FAMP and CDA.

FAMP in Solid Tumours (Table 1)

Five phase I clinical studies were performed in the early eighties among 155 patients and one clinical response was observed in a patient with lung cancer [6-10]. During the following phase II studies, clinical responses were reported in one patient with advanced head and neck cancer [11], one patient with advanced breast cancer [12] and one patient with astrocytoma [13]. Further phase II studies performed in lung cancer [14,15], breast cancer [16], ovarian cancer [17,18], colorectal cancer [19, 20], genito-urinary tract cancer [21-24], liver and pancreatic cancer [25,26], soft tissue sarcoma [27], head and neck cancer [28], glioma [29] and melanoma [30], in a total of over 400 patients, failed to identify any responding solid tumour. The schedule of administration was usually 5-daily intravenous injection at doses varying between 18 and 40 mg/m2/d. In one responding patient FAMP was administered by continuous 24-hour intravenous infusion for 5 days [12]. The main toxicity was myelosuppression but 2 cases of fatal renal failure have been reported [26].

CDA in Solid Tumours (Table 2)

No phase I and II studies with CDA have been performed according to the classic standards despite the early identification of high activity in haematologiclal malignancies [31]. Furthermore, CDA was not available for investigators out of the Scripps Research Institute until recently. Proper phase I studies are simply lacking and there are only two reported phase II studies in solid tumours. In the first study, 12 patients with colorectal cancer and 2 patients with soft tissue sarcoma received CDA at escalating doses but no antitumour activity was seen [32]. In the second study, 7 patients with astrocytoma, 12 with melanoma and 2 with renal cell carcinoma were treated; 2 patients with astrocytoma showed partial responses [33]. On the whole, 35 patients with various solid tumours received CDA with little

Table 1. Fludarabine monophosphate studies in solid tumours

Tumour	Number of patients	Number of responses	Author (ref)
Lung (phase I)	13	1	Hutton et al. [6]
Breast	15	0	Carpenter et al. [16]
NSCLC	23	0	Weiss et al. [14]
Ovary	29	0	Kavanagh et al. [17]
Head & neck	25	1	Weiss et al. [11]
Colorectum	22	0	Harvey et al. [19]
Hepatoma	19	0	Harvey et al. [25]
STS	23	0	Pazdur et al. [27]
Renal cell	36	0	Balducci et al. [21]
SCLC	11	0	Rainey et al. [15]
Ovary	21	0	Von Hoff et al. [18]
Colorectum	21	0	Ajani et al. [20]
Glioma	15	0	Cascino et al. [29]
Breast	18	1	Mitelman et al. [12]
Renal cell	18	0	Shevrin et al. [22]
Head & neck	13	0	Mitelman et al. [28]
Cervix	21	0	Von Hoff et al. [23]
Endometrium	20	0	Von Hoff et al. [24]
Melanoma	27	0	Kish et al. [30]
CNS	23	1	Taylor et al. [13]
Pancreas	20	0	Kilton et al. [26]
Total	**433**	**4**	

SCLC = small cell lung carcinoma   NSCLC = non-small cell lung carcinoma
STS = soft tissue sarcoma   CNS = central nervous system

Table 2. Cladribine studies in solid tumours

Tumour	Number of patients	Number of responses	Author (ref)
Colorectal	12	0	Weiss et al. [32]
STS	2	0	Weiss et al. [32]
Astrocytoma	7	2	Saven et al. [33]
Renal cell	2	0	Saven et al. [33]
Melanoma	12	0	Saven et al. [33]
Total	**35**	**2**	

indication of any useful activity. CDA was administered by continuous intravenous infusion over 5 or 7 days at doses ranging between 3.25 and 6.5 mg/m^2/d. Further escalation was not possible because of myelosuppression; an additional side-effect was neurotoxicity [33].

Discussion

FAMP and CDA seem to be inactive in the managment of non-haematological tumours. However, it is too early to draw any final conclusions regarding this apparent absence of activity. Other schedules of administration as well as combination with other agents and radiotherapy deserve further testing. Modulation of the activating enzyme dCTk and of the catabolic enzyme 5'-NT should also be considered. Finally, since myelosuppression is the dose-limiting toxicity, administration of the colony-stimulating growth factors could be of great help in optimising phase II studies.

REFERENCES

1 Grever M, Leiby J, Kraut E et al: A comprehensive phase I and II clinical investigation of fludarabine phosphate. Semin Oncol 1990 (17):39-48
2 Beutler E: Cladribine (2-chlorodeoxyadenosine). Lancet 1992 (340):952-956
3 Gandhi V, Estey E, Keating MJ, Plunkett W: Fludarabine potentiates metabolism of cytarabine in patients with acute myelogenous leukemia during therapy. J Clin Oncol 1993 (11):116-124
4 Kawasaki K, Carrera CJ, Piro LD et al: Relationship of deoxycytidine kinase and cytoplasmic 5'-nucleotidase to the chemotherapeutic efficacy of 2-chlorodeoxyadenosine. Blood 1993 (81): 597-601
5 Robertson LE, Chubb S, Meyn RE et al: Induction of apoptotic cell death in chronic lymphocytic leukemia by 2-chloro-2'-deoxyadenosine and 9-ß-D-arabinosyl-2-fluoroadenine. Blood 1993 (81):143-150
6 Hutton JJ, Von DD, Kuhn T et al: Phase I clinical investigation of 9-ß-D-arabinofuranosyl-2-fluoroadenine 5'-monophosphate (NSC312887), a new purine antimetabolite. Cancer Res 1984 (44):4183-4186
7 Grever MR, Kraut EH, Neidhart JA et al: 2-Fluoro-ara-AMP. A phase I clinical investigation. Invest New Drugs 1984 (2):116
8 Leiby JM, Grever MR, Staubus AE et al: Phase I clinical investigation of fludarabine phosphate by a loading dose and continuous infusion schedule. JNCI 1988 (80):447-449
9 Casper ES, Mittleman A, Kelson J et al: Phase I clinical trial of fludarabine phosphate (F-ara-AMP). Cancer Chemother Pharmacol 1985 (15):233-235
10 Kavanagh JJ, Krakoff IH, Bodey GP: Phase I study of fludarabine (2-fluoro-ara-AMP). Eur J Cancer Clin Oncol 1985 (21):1009-1011
11 Weiss GB, Metch B, von Hoff DD et al: Phase II trial of fludarabine phosphate in patients with head and neck cancer. A Southwest Oncology Group study. Cancer Treat Rep 1987 (71):1313-1314
12 Mittelman A, Ashikari R, Ahmed T et al: Phase II trial of fludarabine phosphate (F-ara-AMP) in patients with advanced breast cancer. Cancer Chemother Pharmacol 1988 (22):63-64
13 Taylor SA, Crowley J, Vogel FS et al: Phase II evaluation of fludarabine phosphate in patients with central nervous system tumors. Invest New Drugs 1991 (9):195-197
14 Weiss GR, Crowley J, von Hoff DD et al: Phase II study of fludarabine phosphate for the treatment of advanced non-small cell carcinoma of the lung. A Southwest Oncology Group study. Cancer Treat Rep 1986 (70):1123-1124
15 Rainey JM, Hill JB, Crowley J: Evaluation of fludarabine phosphate in small cell carcinoma. A Southwest Oncology Group study. Invest New Drugs 1988 (6):45-46
16 Carpenter JT, Vogel CL, Wang G, Raney M: Phase II evaluation of fludarabine in patients with metastatic breast cancer. A Southeastern Cancer Study Group trial. Cancer Treat Rep 1986 (70): 1235-1236
17 Kavanagh JJ, Stringer CA, Copeland LJ et al: Phase II trial of fludarabine in patients with epithelial ovarian cancer. Cancer Treat Rep 1986 (70):425-426
18 Von Hoff DD, Kronmal R, O'Toole RV et al: Phase II study of fludarabine phosphate (NSC-312887) in patients with advanced ovarian cancer. A Southwest Oncology Group study. Am J Clin Oncol 1988 (11):146-148
19 Harvey WH, Fleming TR, von Hoff DD et al: Phase II trial of fludarabine phosphate in previously untreated patients with colorectal carcinoma. A Southwest Oncology Group study. Cancer Treat Rep 1987 (71):1319-1320
20 Ajani JA, Abbruzzese JL, Faintuch JS et al: Phase II study of fludarabine phosphate in patients with advanced colorectal carcinoma. Invest New Drugs 1988 (6):47-50
21 Balducci L, Blumenstein B, von Hoff DD et al: Evaluation of fludarabine phosphate in renal cell carcinoma. A Southwest Oncology Group study. Cancer Treat Rep 1987 (71):543-544
22 Shevrin DH, Lad TE, Kilton LJ et al: Phase II trial of fludarabine phosphate in advanced renal cell carcinoma. An Illinois Cancer Council study. Invest New Drugs 1989 (7):251-253
23 Von Hoff DD, Green S, Surwit EA et al: Phase II study of fludarabine phosphate (NSC 312887) in patients with advanced cervical cancer. A Southwest Oncology Group study. Am J Clin Oncol 1990 (13):433-435
24 Von Hoff DD, Green S, Surwit EA et al: Phase II study of fludarabine phosphate (NSC-312887) in patients with advanced endometrial cancer. A Southwest Oncology Group study. Am J Clin Oncol 1991 (14):193-194
25 Harvey WH, Fleming TR, Beltran G et al: Phase II study of fludarabine phosphate in previously untreated patients with hepatoma. A Southwest Oncology Group study. Cancer Treat Rep 1987 (71): 1111-1112
26 Kilton LJ, Benson AB, Greenberg A et al: Phase II trial of fludarabine phosphate for adenocarcioma of the pancreas. Invest New Drugs 1992 (10):291-294
27 Pazdur R, Samson MK, Baker LH: Fludarabine phosphate. Phase II evaluation in advanced soft-tissue sarcomas. Am J Clin Oncol 1987 (10):341-343

28 Mitelman A, Savona S, Puccio C et al: Phase II trial of fludarabine phosphate (F-Ara-AMP) in patients with advanced head and neck cancer. Invest New Drugs 1990 (8): 565-567

29 Cascino T, Brown LD, Morton RF et al: Evaluation of fludarabine phosphate in patients with recurrent glioma. Am J Clin Oncol 1988 (11):586-588

30 Kish JA, Kopecky K, Samson MK et al: Evaluation of fludarabine phosphate in malignant melanoma. A Southwest Oncology Group study. Invest New Drugs 1991 (9):105-108

31 Carson DA, Wasson DB, Lamon J, Beutler E: A potent new anti-lymphocyte agent: 2-chlorodeoxyadenosine. Blood 1982 (60):161 (abstract)

32 Weiss G, Kuhn J, Irvin R et al: Phase I trial of 2-chlorodeoxyadenosine (2-CDA) by 120-hour infusion for solid cancers. Proc ASCO 1993 (12): 455 (abstract)

33 Saven A, Kawasaki H, Carrera C et al: 2-Chlorodeoxyadenosine dose escalation in nonhematologic malignancies. J Clin Oncol 1993 (11):671-678

Advanced Breast Cancer: Experience with Gemcitabine

Kurt Possinger [1], James Carmichael [2], Philip Phillip [3], Maria Beykirch [4], Helen Kerr [3], Jackie Walling [5] and Adrian L. Harris [3]

1 Medizinische Klinik II, Universitätsklinikum Charité, Schumannstrasse 20/21, 10 117 Berlin, Germany
2 Nottingham General Hospital, Nottingham, United Kingdom
3 ICRF Clinical Oncology Unit, Churchill Hospital, Oxford OX3 7LF, United Kingdom
4 Medizinische Klinik III, Klinikum Großhadern, Marchionistrasse 15, 81366 Munich, Germany
3 Lilly Industries Ltd., Dextra Court, Chapel Hill, Basingstoke Hants RG21 2SY, United Kingdom

In metastatic breast cancer, cure is beyond our reach at present. Endocrine and cytotoxic therapies offer the most useful forms of treatment. Combination chemotherapy can induce response rates of more than 50%; however, there is no good evidence that such treatment significantly prolongs survival.

Therefore we aim for symptomatic palliation, increased subjective well-being and preservation of physical ability. Under this aspect there is a clear need for the development of new anticancer drugs with reliable activity and low systemic toxicity.

Gemcitabine, a new antimetabolite, seems to be active in several solid tumours and possibly in malignant lymphomas and leukaemias.

Two breast cancer studies with gemcitabine have been completed, one in Europe and the other in the US. These studies have shown disparate results.

US Study

The US study was designed as a multicentre trial. Gemcitabine was administered intravenously once a week for 3 weeks, followed by a 1-week rest period. The initial dose of gemcitabine was 800 mg/m^2, and subsequent doses were modified on the basis of haematological and non-haematological toxicity.

With the exception of one patient who was chemotherapy naive, gemcitabine was given as second or third-line palliative cytotoxic therapy.

Twenty-one patients were enrolled, 20 received at least one dose of gemcitabine. Only 14 patients were evaluable for efficacy assessment. There were no responses.

Although the average dose intensity was 662 mg/m^2, this figure needs to be viewed in the light of the observation that the range of administered cycles was 1 to 14 but the median was only 2. However, 1 patient received 14 cycles with the majority of treatment being given at the escalated level of 1250 mg/m^2. Therefore the doses received by this patient have had a substantial effect on the average dose intensity.

There were significant numbers of dose omissions and reductions in the study: overall, 11.9% of all injections were omitted and 31.1% were reduced. The reasons for dose reductions were not specified.

European Study

In Europe patients were recruited to a 2-centre breast cancer study conducted jointly by the Churchill Hospital, Oxford, U.K. and the Klinikum Großhadern, Munich, Germany. Gemcitabine was administered on an outpatient basis.

A dose of 800 mg/m^2 was given as a 30-minute i.v. infusion once weekly for 3 weeks followed by a week of rest. This constituted one course of chemotherapy. Drug dose was reduced by 50% for grade 2 myelosuppression.

Toxicity was scored monthly using WHO criteria, and the clinical response was initially as-

Table 1. Patient characteristics

Total number of patients	44
Age (years)	
median	54.5
mean	53.81
range	32 - 77
Performance status	
0	14
1	25
2	5
Menopausal status	
pre	9
peri	4
post	31
Histology	
ductal	35
lobular	3
adeno	5
mixed	1
Differentiation	
poor	15
moderate	7
well	2
unknown	20
Spread	
loco-regional	4
metastatic	40

Table 2. Haematological toxicity in %

WHO grade	0	1	2	3	4
Haemoglobin	47.7	45.5	4.5	2.3	0
Leukocytes	18.2	18.2	54.5	6.8	2.3
Segmented neutrophils	25.6	16.3	27.9	23.2	7.0
Platelets	86.4	6.8	2.3	2.3	2.2

sessed using WHO criteria following 2 courses of chemotherapy.

Forty-four patients with advanced breast cancer (locoregional recurrence or metastatic disease) with measurable disease in a previously unirradiated area were admitted to the study. Patients were allowed a maximum of one regimen of chemotherapy as adjuvant treatment or for advanced disease. They had to be aged between 18 and 75 years with a WHO performance status of ≤2, serum creatinine <150 mmol/l, serum bilirubin less than twice normal, and ALT/AST less than 3 times normal.

Patients with endocrine or radiotherapy in the 4 weeks before the start of the study, with symptomatic involvement of the central nervous system, concomitant cytotoxic, hormonal treatment, immunotherapy, corticosteroids (except corticosteroid antiemetics and oral contraceptives) or experimental agents were excluded. The patient characteristics are summarised in Table 1.

Of the 44 patients entered in the study, 31 were evaluable for efficacy as defined by the protocol. All 13 non-evaluable patients had received less than the 56 days of treatment required for response definition by the protocol. Among the 31 protocol-qualified patients, 3 achieved a complete response and 7 a partial response, resulting in an overall response rate of 32.3% (95% confidence interval: 16.7-51.4). Responses were seen in soft tissue (breast, lymph nodes) and in 4 patients with liver metastases. Five responders had received previous chemotherapy, 3 had received up to 3 hormonal therapies, and 2 were chemotherapy naive. The duration of response ranged from 4 months to 18 months. The median overall survival times were 18.6 months for responders and 8.6 months for non-responders. The response in patients with the intention to treat was 25% (95% CI: 12.7-41.2). All responses were confirmed by an independent Oncology Review Board.

There were a number of symptomatic benefits including decreased analgesic consumption (median duration of improvement 11.6 weeks), increased performance status (median duration 4 weeks), and decreased pain score (median duration 18 weeks).

Only 5% of injections were omitted (more than half of these because of progressive disease), 2% were delayed, and 12% were reduced (all reductions due to protocol-mandated leukopenia).

The WHO toxicity grades for laboratory parameters are given in Tables 2 and 3. Haematological toxicity was generally mild; in particular very little platelet toxicity was observed, 86.4% of patients having no abnormal platelet count. Although the most sensitive indicator of myelosuppression was neutropenia, with WHO toxicity grades 3 and 4 of 23.3% and 7.0%, respectively, the incidence of infection

Table 3. Laboratory values in %

WHO-Grade	0	1	2	3	4
Bilirubin	97.7	2.3	0	0	0
Aspartate transaminase	25.0	36.4	29.5	6.8	2.3
Alanine transaminase	45.5	36.4	0	18.2	0
Alkaline phosphatase	65.9	20.5	13.6	0	0
Urea	81.0	19.0	0	0	0
Creatinine	100	0	0	0	0
Proteinuria	55.8	34.9	9.3	0	0
Haematuria	62.8	20.9	16.3	0	0

Table 4. Non-haematological toxicity in %

WHO-Grade	0	1	2	3	4
Infection	90.9	4.5	2.3	0	2.3
Fever	70.5	20.5	9.0	0	0
Hair loss	77.2	9.1	11.4	2.3	0
Consciousness	54.5	25.0	18.2	2.3	0
Pulmonary	86.4	6.8	6.8	0	0
Allergic	97.7	0	0	2.3	0
Cutaneous	75.0	18.2	4.5	2.3	0
Peripheral neurotoxicity	97.7	2.3	0	0	0
Nausea /vomiting	38.6	27.3	6.8	25.0	2.3
Oral	88.7	4.5	6.8	0	0
Diarrhoea	86.4	4.5	9.1	0	0
Constipation	93.2	6.8	0	0	0

associated with this level of neutropenia was very low.

Liver toxicity was minimal, and in the majority of patients displaying abnormal enzyme levels, toxicity was mild. Only one patient discontinued treatment due to liver toxicity.

The WHO toxicity grades for symptomatic toxicity are given in Table 4. The only WHO grade 4 symptomatic toxicities were infection (2.3%) and nausea and vomiting (2%). WHO grade 3 toxicities were few but included nausea and vomiting (25%), flu-like symptoms (2.3%), hair loss (2.3%), and cutaneous symptoms (2.3%). The incidence of fever was low. Peripheral oedema was reported in 9.1% of patients and oedema in 4.5%.

Conclusion

In the European study, gemcitabine has been shown to be active in advanced breast cancer with an independently validated response rate of 32.3% (95% CI: 16.7-51.4). There were 3 complete responses and 7 partial responses. In the European and the US studies gemcitabine toxicity was mild and predominantly non-haematological. The schedule, once a week for 3 weeks followed by a week of rest, was well tolerated on an outpatient basis. The toxicity profile of gemcitabine does not overlap significantly with other cytotoxic agents used in breast cancer. Gemcitabine is therefore a logical choice for trials in combination with other agents used against breast cancer.

Gemcitabine in Ovarian Cancer

Jan P. Neijt [1] and Birthe Lund [2]

1   Department of Internal Medicine, Section of Oncology, Utrecht University Hospital, Heidelberglaan 100,
    3584 CX Utrecht, The Netherlands
2   Department of Oncology, Rigshospitalet, 9, Blegdamsvej, 2100 Copenhagen, Denmark

In the last decade many therapeutic options have been investigated for ovarian cancer. Most of them have not led to results with implications for standard practice. It is obvious that new drugs are needed to improve the results in advanced disease. Recently the introduction of taxanes in the treatment of ovarian cancer has engendered hope that treatment may further improve. Gemcitabine is another promising candidate to be added to the list of drugs active in ovarian cancer. The drug showed activity in a group of patients not very likely to respond. In this review we will first discuss the factors that determine the outcome of phase II studies, such as the initial treatment and previous second-line treatment, and then we will take a closer look at the results obtained with gemcitabine.

Current Initial and Second-Line Treatment

At present the use of a combination of agents including platinum is recommended as initial treatment for ovarian cancer because platinum-based chemotherapy gives superior response rates, progression-free survival and probably also long-term survival. In a recent consensus meeting treatment with either cyclophosphamide 750 mg/m^2 plus cisplatin 75 mg/m^2 every 3 weeks (CP) or cyclophosphamide 500 mg/m^2 plus doxorubicin 50 mg/m^2 plus cisplatinum 50 mg/m^2 every 3 weeks was accepted as standard therapy [1]. Carboplatin, and more recently paclitaxel (taxol), are the two drugs competing to be incorporated in the standard treatment: carboplatin to replace cisplatin, paclitaxel to replace cyclophosphamide. It is not generally accepted that carboplatin can replace cisplatin in the initial treatment [2]. Comparative trials suggest that carboplatin in a myelotoxic combination may lead to inferior results compared to cisplatin in the same combination. Adjusting the dose of carboplatin or delaying treatment cycles to permit recovery of leukocytes and platelets may influence the survival results negatively. Both considerations led the participants of the consensus meeting to conclude that carboplatin-based therapy is an acceptable choice for patients with suboptimal stage III and stage IV ovarian cancer, but not for patients with good prognostic features; cisplatin-based therapy is the preferred treatment in the latter group.

Paclitaxel is after many years the first drug with promising activity. In 1993 the Gynecologic Oncology Group (GOG) in the USA presented the results with this drug used in the frontline setting. In the CP combination cyclophosphamide was replaced by paclitaxel (135 mg/m^2 over 24 hours) and compared with CP. The paclitaxel combination resulted in better response rates and, more importantly, in an improvement in progression-free survival and overall survival [3,4]. The integration of paclitaxel in the standard treatment of ovarian cancer has been criticised because of the inconvenience of the 24-hour administration schedule, the side-effects of paclitaxel plus cisplatin and the expense. A confirmatory trial is now planned by the EORTC in collaboration with the National Cancer Institute of Canada Clinical Trials Group (NCIC-CTG).

At present most centres in Europe agree on a combination of cisplatin and cyclophosphamide as standard treatment. At least 6 treatment courses should be planned. Patients who

Table 1. Variable response rates of phase II drugs used in ovarian cancer

Phase II drugs	Response rates	Reference
Mitoxantrone	0 - 28	Hilgers, 1984 [5]
Cisplatin	15 - 20	Thigpen, 1985 [6]
Carboplatin	8 - 32	Eisenhauer, 1990 [7]
Teniposide	0 - 40	Muggia, 1991 [8]
Ifosfamide	12 - 22	Thigpen,1993 [9]
Hexamethylmelamine	10 - 20	Thigpen,1993
Taxol	20 - 50	Rowinsky, 1992 [10]

reach a clinically complete remission including normal CA 125 levels receive 3 additional cycles of chemotherapy, after which no further chemotherapy seems warranted. In patients with a partial remission treatment can be continued as long as the tumour is not progressive. For those with stable, non-resectable tumours or disease progression, treatment with a new drug in a phase II study can be considered.

The Selection of Patients for Phase II Studies

The results obtained with phase II drugs in ovarian cancer vary widely. As presented in Table 1 the problem is also encountered in the more recent studies with paclitaxel. These variations in response rates are a consequence of the variation in patient populations entered intc these studies. Several prognostic factors other than the efficacy of the phase II drugs determine the final response rate. Blackledge et al. performed an analysis of 5 phase II studies with a total of 93 patients to determine whether factors other than the efficacy of phase II drugs affected response [11]. In the multivariate analysis, only 2 factors were shown to be of importance in determining whether a patient will respond in a phase II study: 1) the interval between previous therapy and entry into the phase II study, and 2) the FIGO stage of the patient. The importance of the interval was emphasised by the fact that the response rate of those patients who progressed on primary treatment and received the phase II therapy within 6 months of completing primary treatment was very low (5 out of 50: 10%). However, those who had an interval greater than 20 months between previous therapy and the phase II treatment responded in 90% of the cases (19 out of 21). A similar study was performed by Markman et al. [12]. To determine the incidence of secondary responses to platinum-based therapy in patients previously treated with cisplatin, they undertook a retrospective review of 82 patients with a cisplatin-free interval of more than 4 months between the completion of their first regimen and the institution of a second cisplatin/carboplatin treatment. Of the 72 evaluable patients 43% responded. The overall response rates based on duration of cisplatin-free interval were: 5 to 12 months, 27%; 13 to 24 months, 33%; and more than 24 months, 59%. Patients without any treatment for more than 24 months experienced a 77% (17 out of 22) response rate. The results of the above studies and of 2 more studies looking for variables predicting time to progression in second-line treatment are summarised in Table 2.

The data indicate that patients with recurrent disease can benefit by second-line treatment. In general the effect of this treatment is dependent on the patient characteristics at the start of treatment. The variables mentioned in Table 2 suggest that patients with a long interval from the chemotherapy, small bulk of disease, serous cell type, and few sites of disease have better chances of responding to a phase II drug or retreatment with cisplatinum. On the contrary patients who had progressive disease during platinum therapy (a very short interval) and larger tumour masses are unlikely to benefit from retreatment or phase II drugs.

Table 2. Prognostic factors associated with a poor prognosis in recurrent advanced ovarian cancer from multivariate analysis [11,13-15]

Variables at the time of relapse associated with a low response rate	Variables at the time of relapse associated with a short time to progression
Bulk of disease > 5 cm	Poor performance status
Cell type other than serous	Interval since last chemotherapy < 6 months
Lower than normal haemoglobin	Cell type other than serous
Interval since last chemotherapy < 6 months	Large number of sites of disease
FIGO stage IV	High serum CA 125 level

Results with Gemcitabine in Second Line

Gemcitabine (2',2'-difluorodeoxycytidine) is a pyrimidine antimetabolite developed as a deoxycytidine analogue [16]. The drug shows a close resemblance to cytosine-arabinoside. In order to assess the activity of gemcitabine in ovarian carcinoma and to characterise the toxicity of the compound, a multicentre phase II study was performed by Lund and coworkers in Denmark [17]. In this study patients were admitted with advanced epithelial ovarian cancer who had received a maximum of 2 prior treatment regimens. Retreatment with the same regimen and substitution of cisplatinum with carboplatin or *vice versa* because of toxicity were considered as one treatment regimen. All patients had measurable disease and a WHO performance status of 2 or less. Patients received gemcitabine 800 mg/m^2, given as a 30 min i.v. infusion on a weekly basis, for 3 consecutive weeks, followed by a fourth week of rest. Dose escalation up to a maximum of 1200 mg/m^2 was allowed. Postponement for 3 weeks or more due to toxicity was a reason for discontinuation of treatment. Response to therapy was assessed every other course by pelvic examination and ultrasound or CT-scans. All response data were reviewed independently by experts not involved in the study.

A total of 51 patients entered the study with 50 patients being eligible. The majority of the patients had bulky disease and all patients had received prior platinum containing combination chemotherapy. Twenty percent of the patients had a complete response and 38% a partial response to prior first-line therapy. A total of 42 patients were evaluable for response. Eight patients (19%; 95% confidence limits 9-34%) achieved a partial response. Median response duration was 8.1 months (range 4.4 to 12.5 months). In Table 3 the prognostic characteristics of these responders to gemcitabine are summarised. It is obvious from this table that all responders had bad prognostic features and a poor chance of responding to gemcitabine as second-line treatment.

Treatment with gemcitabine was very well tolerated. Nausea and vomiting, grade III, occurred only in 6 patients and no hair loss was observed. Specific treatment-related non-haematological side-effects consisted of transient proteinuria, haematuria and an increase in transaminases. One patient developed dose limiting cutaneous toxicity, grade II, and 3 patients showed an increase in serum creatinine. This was dose limiting in one patient. Four patients experienced treatment-related dyspnoea. A flu-like syndrome was observed in 14 patients. This occurred a few hours after the injection of gemcitabine and could last for 24 hours. Asthenia was observed in 23 patients and

Table 3. Variables associated with 8 gemcitabine responders

Variable	Number of patients
< 6 Months since last chemotherapy	8
Progressive while on platinum therapy	7
Bulk of disease > 5 cm	5
FIGO Stage IV	5
Poorly/undifferentiated tumour	6
Best previous response complete remission	1
Best previous response partial remission	3

caused dose reduction in one. Six patients experienced treatment-related myalgia.

A total of 184 courses of gemcitabine was given. The majority of injections were given as assigned, and in 9% the dose was escalated. Leukopenia and thrombocytopenia were the main reasons for dose omissions (27% and 14%, respectively) and for dose reductions (37% and 21%, respectively).

Discussion

Although further research is needed, gemcitabine appears to be an interesting new drug in ovarian cancer. Many other new drugs have been tested in the last decade in phase II studies for ovarian cancer. The results of these studies are difficult to interpret because of differences in the characteristics of the patients admitted to these phase II studies. So far only few drugs have shown clear activity in patients with progressive disease during previous platinum treatment and with unfavourable prognostic characteristics: paclitaxel (taxol) [18], docetaxel (taxotere) [19], etoposide (VP16) [20], and gemcitabine.

Paclitaxel (taxol), now commercially available, was tested in more than 1000 patients who all were platinum refractory [21]. In this study patients with platinum-refractory ovarian cancer who had received at least 3 prior chemotherapy regimens were treated with paclitaxel 135 mg/m^2 administered as a 24-hour continuous infusion, every 3 weeks. The objective response rate was 22% (4% complete responses, 18% partial responses with a 95% confidence interval for overall response of 19-25%). The median time to progression from treatment was 7.8 months in responding patients. It can be noted from these data that paclitaxel has activity in women with platinum-refractory ovarian cancer. For this reason the drug is now moved to the front line. Comparing the results obtained with paclitaxel to those presented in the phase II study of Lund et al., the latter are encouraging. The 19% response rate achieved with gemcitabine with a median response duration of 8.1 months is comparable to the results obtained with taxol. Activity of gemcitabine was also observed in a very small American phase II study in previously treated patients. Two out of 7 patients responded in this study. Response assessment was only based on the decline of the level of the tumour marker CA 125. Unfortunately, information regarding prior treatment in the two responders was not available [22].

The gemcitabine data indicate that gemcitabine may be non cross-resistant to platinum. One may conclude that gemcitabine is well tolerated and has activity in platinum-resistant disease. More studies are needed to confirm the results obtained and to assess the activity of gemcitabine in untreated ovarian cancer with unfavourable features.

REFERENCES

1   Consensus group in alphabetical order: Allen DG, Baak J, Belpomme D, Berek JS, Bertelsen K, ten Bokkel Huinink WW, van der Burg MEL, Calvert AH, Conte PF, Dauplat J, Eisenhauer EA, Favalli G, Hacker NF, Hamilton TC, Hansen HH, Hansen M, van Houwelingen HC, Kaye SB, Levin L, Lund B, Neijt JP, Ozols RF, Piccart MJ, Rustin GJS, Sessa C, Soutter WP, Thigpen JT, Tropé C, Vermorken JB, and De Vries EGE: Advanced epithelial ovarian cancer. 1993 Consensus statements. Ann Oncol 1993 (4):83-89

2   Vermorken JB, Ten Bokkel Huinink WW, Eisenhauer EA, Favalli G, Belpomme D, Conte PF, Kaye SB: Carboplatin versus cisplatin. Ann Oncol 1993 (4):41-48

3   Williams SD for the Gynecological Oncology Group: Stage III trial comparing cisplatin/cyclophosphamide with cisplatin/paclitaxel in advanced ovarian cancer. In: Taxol (paclitaxel), a Novel Advance in Chemotherapy. Symposium program and abstracts. Amsterdam, the Netherlands, October 13 1993, p 22

4   McGuire WP, Hoskins WJ, MF Brady, PR Kucera, Look KY, Padridge EE, Davidson M: A phase III trial comparing cisplatin/cytoxan (PC) and cisplatin/taxol (PT) in advanced ovarian cancer (AOC). Proceedings of ASCO 1993 (12):255

5   Hilgers RD, Rivkin SE, Von Hoff DD, Alberts DS: Mitoxantrone in epithelial carcinoma of the ovary. A Southwest Oncology Group study. Am J Clin Oncol 1984 7(5):499-501

6   Thigpen T and Blessing JA: Current therapy of ovarian carcinoma: an overview. Semin-Oncol 1985 (12 Suppl 4):47-52

7   Eisenhauer EA, Swenerton KD, Sturgeon JFG, Fine S, O'Reilly SEO, Canetta R: Carboplatin therapy for recurrent ovarian carcinoma: National Cancer Institute of Canada experience and a review of the literature. In: Bunn PA, Canetta R, Ozols RF, Rozencweig M (eds) Carboplatin (JM-8). Current Perspectives and Future Directions. WB Saunders Co, Harcourt Brace Jovanovich, Inc, Philadelphia 1990 pp 133-140

8   Muggia FM and Russell CA: New chemotherapies for ovarian cancer. Systemic and intraperitoneal podophyllotoxins. Cancer 1991 (67 Suppl 1):225-230

9   Thigpen JT, Vance RB, Khansur T: Second-line chemotherapy for recurrent carcinoma of the ovary. Cancer 1993 (71 Suppl 4): 1559-1564

10 Rowinsky EK, Onetto N, Canetta RM, Arbuck SG: Taxol: the first of the taxanes. An important new class of antitumor agents. Sem Oncol 1992 (19):646-662

11 Blackledge G, Lawton F, Redman C et al: Response of patients in phase II studies of chemotherapy in ovarian cancer: implications for patient treatment and the design of phase II trials. Br J Cancer 1989 (59):650-653

12 Markman M, Rothman R, Hakes T et al: Second-line platinum therapy in patients with ovarian cancer previously treated with cisplatin. J Clin Oncol 1991 (9):389-393

13 Eisenhauer EA, Ten Bokkel Huinink WW, Swenerton KD, Gianni L, Myles J, Van der Burg MEL, Kerr L, Vermorken JB, Buser K, Colombo N, Bacon M, Santabárbara P, Onetto N, Winograd B, Canetta R: European-Canadian randomized trial of taxol in relapsed ovarian cancer: High vs low dose and long vs short infusion. 1994 (submitted)

14 Hoskins PJ, O'Reilly SE, Swenerton KD: The 'failure free interval' defines the likelihood of resistance to carboplatin in patients with advanced epithelial ovarian cancer previously treated with cisplatin: relevance to therapy and new drug testing. Int J Gynecol Cancer 1991 (1):205-208

15 Makar AP, Kristensen GB, Bormer OP, Trope CG: Is serum CA 125 at the time of relapse a prognostic indicator for further survival prognosis in patients with ovarian cancer? Gynecol Oncol 1993 (49):3-7

16 Lund B, Kristjansen PEG, Hansen HH: Clinical and preclinical activity of 2'2'-difluorodeoxycytidine (gemcitabine). Cancer Treat Rev 1993 (19):45-55

17 Lund B, Hansen OP, Theilade K, Hansen M, Neijt JP: Phase II study of gemcitabine (2',2',-difluorodeoxycytidine) in previously treated ovarian cancer. 1994 (submitted)

18 Hansen HH, Eisenhauer EA, Hansen M, Neijt JP, Piccart MJ, Bertelsen K, Levin L, Lund B: New cytotoxic drugs in ovarian cancer. Ann Oncol 1993 (4):63-70

19 Aapro M, Pujade-Lauraine E, Lhomme C, Lentz M-A, le Bail N, Fumoleau P, Chevallier B: Phase II study of Taxotere™ (T) in ovarian cancer. EORTC: Clinical Screening Group (CSG). Proc Am Soc Cancer Clin Oncol 1993 (12):809

20 Hoskins PJ, Swenerton KD: Oral etoposide is active against platinum-resistant ovarian cancer. J Clin Oncol 1994 (12):60-63

21 Trimble EL, Adams JD, Vena D et al: Paclitaxel for platinum-refractory ovarian cancer: Results from the first 1000 patients registered to National Cancer Institute Treatment Referral Center 9103. J Clin Oncol 1993 (12):2405-2410

22 Morgan-Ihrig C, Lembersky B, Christopherson W, Tarassoff P: A phase II elevation of difluorodeoxycytidine (dFdC) in advanced stage refractory ovarian cancer. Proc Am Soc Clin Oncol 1991 (10):196

Gemcitabine Therapy in Non-Small Cell Lung Cancer: A Review

Thierry Le Chevalier

Comité de Pathologie Thoracique, Institut Gustave Roussy, Rue Camille Desmoulins, 94805 Villejuif Cedex, France

The treatment of advanced non-small cell lung cancer (NSCLC) has not made very significant progress with regard to response rates and survival in the last decade. Few single agents have, in large studies, achieved response rates of more than 15%, while combination treatment gives response rates of 25% to 35% [1-4]. Several randomised studies comparing chemotherapy with best supportive care have yielded predominantly slightly favourable results for chemotherapy [5]. Two recent meta-analyses of the literature indicated a significant but modest survival advantage for the use of platinum-containing combination treatment compared with best supportive care [6,7].

A significant concern with many of these treatment regimens has been the side-effect profile demonstrated by the chemotherapy regimen when viewed against the modest gains in overall survival. As a result, the benefit to patients has been debated despite the suggestion that patients have diminished disease-related symptoms if they respond to chemotherapy. More recently, however, this nihilistic approach has been questioned. While it is necessary to be mindful of the toxicity imposed upon patients by the administration of chemotherapy, there is mounting evidence indicating that chemotherapy may indeed be capable of palliation in this disease [8]. It is therefore important that the assessment of new chemotherapeutic agents for NSCLC should consider not only potential gains in objective efficacy parameters but also the role in palliation of distressing symptoms, and should look for demonstrated advantages in toxicity profile.

Gemcitabine is a novel pyrimidine analogue with activity reported against several solid tumours, including breast cancer, ovarian and small cell lung cancer [9-11]. In particular, gem-citabine has been investigated in extensive phase II NSCLC studies. Three such studies are of primary interest, each of them assessing the role of gemcitabine in a phase II setting in patients with locally advanced, inoperable (AJC stage III and IV) NSCLC. Patients were chemotherapy naive, with a performance status between 0 and 2. In each study gemcitabine was administered weekly for 3 weeks with a fourth week of rest. The infusion duration was 30 minutes, in an outpatient setting. It was not necessary to provide specific prophylactic therapy for nausea and vomiting, and the drug was easily administered.

In an initial study by Anderson and coworkers including a total of 82 patients, an objective tumour response of 24% was documented [12]. This study commenced at an initial dose of 800 mg/m^2 but the protocol was subsequently amended to commence at a dose of 1,000 mg/m^2. Approximately half the patients had stage IV disease (48%), while 29% had stage IIIB disease. A total of 16 out of 68 evaluable patients displayed objective evidence of a partial response. There were no complete responses. The median response duration was 7 months, with an overall median survival of 7 months. This study prospectively assessed disease-related symptoms, and documented improvement in performance status (44%) and pain (44%). This was supported by a decrease in analgesic consumption in 21% of patients.

In a follow-up phase II study in which the starting dose was initially 1,000 mg/m^2 and was increased to 1,250 mg/m^2, Abratt and coworkers documented a 20% objective response rate including 2 complete responses [13]. Eighty-four patients were enrolled with 76 evaluable, giving 15 responses. The median survival for the whole group was 9.2 months, comparing favourably with other agents in phase II studies. Significantly, the patient population included 42% stage IV disease and 40.5% stage IIIB. Pretreatment prognostic factors were typical of this type of phase II study. The toxicity profile was favourable, with WHO grade III or IV leukocyte toxicity following approximately 1% of injections and WHO grade III and IV platelet toxicity following less than 0.5% of injections.

In the most recent and extensive NSCLC study performed to date, including 161 enrolled and 151 evaluable patients with adenocarcinoma and squamous cell carcinoma, Gatzemeier and colleagues report an overall response rate of 22% (33 responders including 3 complete responses) [14]. This study population had late stage disease (stage IIIB 31%; stage IV 65%) with a favourable performance status (PS 1, 83%). The starting dose for this study was 1,250 mg/m^2, with no protocol amendments. As in the previous 2 studies, patients had the opportunity of subsequent dose escalation if the first cycle of therapy was well tolerated. The investigators report a median response duration of 7.6 months, and a median survival for the entire population of 8.9 months. Interestingly, this study documented improvement in disease-related symptoms, including pain relief in 31.3% of patients (supported by an objective decrease in analgesic consumption in 27.7% of patients), cough, dyspnoea, haemoptysis, anorexia, somnolence and hoarseness.

Unique in the reporting of all of these studies has been the incorporation of an independent review of all efficacy data. Radiological and clinical data in support of each investigator-determined response was submitted to an experienced panel of oncologists who, after thorough review of the data, determined the validity of the response status claimed. Patients determined by the board not to fulfil the criteria for objective partial or complete response were reclassified appropriately.

All 3 studies demonstrated favourable toxicity profiles. Haematological toxicity was modest, with WHO grade III and IV neutropenia being documented in 20.9% and 5.7% of patients, respectively, for starting doses up to 1,250 mg/m^2 in the largest study. Thrombocytopenia appeared uncommon. Alterations were also seen in transaminase enzymes, with approximately a third of patients displaying WHO grade I toxicity and another third grade II. This appeared of minimal clinical relevance. Gemcitabine administration in this dosing schedule appeared to be associated with the occurrence of vague and ill-defined flu-like symptoms, including myalgia, fever and asthenia. Peripheral oedema was also reported frequently (up to 30%), the aetiology of which has not been determined as yet.

Conclusion

In larger studies a response rate with gemcitabine of around 20% has been obtained in patients with locally advanced or metastatic NSCLC. With its very mild haematological toxicity profile and novel mechanism of action, this drug is of distinct interest for incorporation into combination regimens; this will be the subject of further studies. As a single agent gemcitabine appears likely to have a role in the palliation of disease-related symptoms with an excellent tolerance profile.

REFERENCES

1   Lenzi R, Fossella FV, Lee JS: Systemic treatment of non-small cell lung cancer. Compre Ther 1992 (18):27-30

2   Splinter TAW: Chemotherapy in advanced non-small cell lung cancer. Eur J Cancer 1990 (26):1093-1099

3   Sandler AB, Buzaid AC: Lung cancer: a review of current therapeutic modalities. Lung 1992 (170):249-265

4   Ihde DC: Chemotherapy of lung cancer. N Engl J Med 1992 (327):1434-1441

5   Rapp E, Pater JL, Willan A, Cormier Y, Murray N, Evans WK, Hodson DI, Clark DA, Feld R, Arnold AM, Ayoub JI, Wilson KS, Latreille J, Wierzbicki RF, Hill DP: Chemotherapy can prolong survival in patients with advanced non-small cell lung cancer - report of a Canadian multicenter randomized trial. J Clin Oncol 1988 (6):633-641

6   Souquet PJ, Chauvin F, Boissel JP, Cellerino R, Cormier Y, Ganz PA, Kaasa S, Pater JL, Quoix E, Rapp E, Tumarello D, Williams J, Woods BL, Bernard JP: Polychemotherapy in advanced non-small cell lung cancer: a meta-analysis. Lancet 1993 (342):19-21

7   Grilli R, Oxman AD, Julian JA: Chemotherapy for advanced non-small cell lung cancer: how much benefit is enough? J Clin Oncol 1993 (11):1866-1872

8   Smith IE: Palliative chemotherapy for advanced non-small cell lung cancer. Br Med J 1994 (308):429-430

9   Carmichael J, Possinger K, Philip P, Beykirch M, Kerr H, Walling J, Harris AL: Difluorodeoxycytidine (gemcitabine): a phase II study in patients with advanced breast cancer. ASCO Proceedings 1993 (12):64 #57

10 Lund B, Hansen OP, Theilade K, Hansen M, Neijt JL: Phase II study of gemcitabine in previously platinum treated ovarian cancer patients. An update. ASCO Proceedings 1993 (12):262 #834

11 Eisenhauer E, Cormier Y, Gregg R, Stewart D, Muldal A: Gemcitabine is active in patients with previously untreated extensive small-cell lung cancer. A phase II study of the National Cancer Institute of Canada Clinical Trials Group. ASCO Proceedings 1992 (11):#1043

12 Anderson H et al: Final report accepted by J Clin Oncol

13 Abratt R et al: Final reported accepted by J Clin Oncol

14 Gatzemeier V et al: abstract: accepted for publication, 7th World Lung Conference, Colorado Springs, 1994

Chemotherapy in Advanced Non-Small Cell Lung Cancer. Changes in Performance Status and Tumour-Related Symptoms

Nick Thatcher, Malcolm Ranson and Heather Anderson

CRC Department of Medical Oncology, University of Manchester, Christie Hospital and Wythenshawe Hospital, Manchester M20 4BX, United Kingdom

A very large number of patients are presently dying of advanced non-small cell lung cancer (NSCLC) for whom improvement in chemotherapy is the only realistic possibility of increasing survival. The problem is that relatively few active agents have been identified. Many earlier studies also involved combinations of drugs with minimal antitumour effect. It is not surprising therefore that chemotherapy of NSCLC was and still is considered by some to be of little or of no value.

Nevertheless, a few agents, such as ifosfamide, cisplatin, mitomycin and vindesine, have objective response rates of 15% or more [1]. Gemcitabine, the new pyrimidine antimetabolite, has a comparable response rate of 20% (95% confidence limits 15.7-24.7) taken from the database of 332 evaluable patients with advanced NSCLC entered into 4 separate studies.

On examination of 61 phase II studies of combination chemotherapy in advanced NSCLC, the average objective response rate still was only 31% with rare complete responses, a median survival of 6 to 9 months and a 1-year survival of around 20% [2,3]. Gemcitabine has an objective response rate of 20%, which has been confirmed by an outside review board who examined the scans, radiographs etc. The median survival ranges from 8.1-9.2 months in the 4 single-agent gemcitabine studies and the 1-year survival is 30-40%.

There is little evidence from the randomised trials to date that combination chemotherapy has a very significant survival advantage over the use of single agents [2]. Indeed carboplatin as a single agent used as initial therapy (followed by mitomycin, vinblastine and cisplatin on pro-gression) had a superior survival compared with combination chemotherapy [4]. It is important therefore to recognise single-agent activity of new drugs such as gemcitabine.

Chemotherapy versus Best Supportive Care

It is reasonable to address the important question as to whether chemotherapy offers any advantage over best supportive care in advanced NSCLC. The earliest randomised studies from Oxford [5,6] used drugs which now would be considered ineffective. However, there is evidence from more recent randomised studies that modest survival benefit can be obtained with combination chemotherapy over best supportive care which in some studies included palliative radiotherapy (Table 1) [2,3,7-12]. The large study from Canada later was assessed in terms of cost effectiveness [7,14]. Economic advantage was claimed for patients treated with chemotherapy over the cost incured for patients who received supportive care only [14]. The British Medical Research Council (MRC) is currently undertaking a meta-analysis of 11 randomised trials (8 containing cisplatin) to determine whether the difference in survival with chemotherapy is statistically significant over that of best supportive care. Recently a meta-analysis of 7 trials has been published [15]. However, the difference in median survival time is only a few months (Table 1). Although the difference is small, a subset of advanced disease patients

Table 1. Chemotherapy versus supportive care in locally advanced and metastatic NSCLC

Reference	Regimen	Patient numbers	OR%	Median survival (months) CT v. No CT		% Survival 1 yr CT v. No CT		p value
Cormier '85	MACC	39	35	7.6	2.1	35	6	0.005
Rapp '88	CAP	150	15	6.1	4.2	21	10	0.01
	PV		25	8.1		22		
Ganz '89	PVb	48	22	5.1	3.3	20	10	NS
Woods '90	PV	201	28	6.8	4.3	NR	NR	NS
Buccheri '90	MACC	175	8	8	5	27	17	0.01
Kaasa '91	PE	87	11	5.0	3.8	NR	NR	NS
Cellerino '91	CEP/MEC	128	21	8.5	5	32	23	NS
Quoix '91	PV	49	42	7.1	2.6	NR	NR	<0.001
Leung '92	PE	119	21	12.4	8.7	53	30	0.05
Cartei '93	PMC	102	25	8.5	4.0	38.5	12	<0.0001

CT - chemotherapy
MACC - methotrexate, doxorubicin, cyclophosphamide, CCNU; CAP - cyclophosphamide, doxorubicin, cisplatin; PV - cisplatin, vindesine; PVb - cisplatin, vinblastine; PE - cisplatin, etoposide; CEP - cyclophosphamide, epirubicin, cisplatin alternating with MEC - methotrexate, etoposide, CCNU; PMC - cisplatin, mitomycin, cyclophosphamide
NR - not recorded
NS - not significant, p > 0.05
Modified from references 2,3, 7-13

clearly derive benefit from chemotherapy, but the majority fail to respond. Identifying the characteristics of this subgroup of patients is important. In assessing the value of treatment further, the impact on quality of life, time without symptoms and performance status changes should also be examined.

Performance Status

One of the problems with chemotherapy for advanced NSCLC is the prejudice that patients' performance status and quality of life always deteriorate with chemotherapy. Change in performance status has been described in some studies but this parameter is often disregarded or the data have been impossible to collect [3]. In randomised trials of chemotherapy against best supportive care, no deterioration in performance scores with chemotherapy has been noted in 3 studies [3]. In one phase II study a 48% response was described but there was a fall in performance status which was considered to remove any potential advantage for the majority of patients [16]. Other studies with more complete data demonstrated that in about one third of patients the performance status improved and in another third remained constant (see Table 2) [17-22]. In a recent MRC study of palliative radiotherapy in advanced non-small cell lung cancer, the performance status in terms of physical activity before therapy was as fol-

Table 2. Change in performance status

Reference	Regimen	Patient numbers	OR%	Median survival (months)	Performance % of Pts		
					+	s	-
Thatcher '86	I	48	29	5	37	35	28
Bakker '86	PVdB	28	48	8	1 patient		
Thatcher '88	IC	45	38	7	40	27	33
Cullen '88	MIP	74	56	9	30	61	9
Kris '90	EDAM MV	85	59	12.8	44	40	26
Gurney '91	IM	42	24	7	24	64	12
von Rohr '92	IM Carbo	34	32	11	37	30	33
MRC '91	XRT	369	30	6	40*	-	-
Anderson '93	Gemcitabine	82	23	8.1	31	67	2
All studies	Gemcitabine	332	20	8.1-9.2	52*	-	-

+ = better, s = stable, - = worse
*patients improving from PS 2
I - ifosfamide; PVdB cisplatin, vindesine and bleomycin; C - cyclophosphamide; M - mitomycin C; P - cisplatin;
V - vinblastine; 10 EDAM - methotrexate analogue; Carbo - carboplatin; XRT - radiotherapy
Modified from references 16-24

lows: PS 0 - 8%, PS 1,2 - 81%, PS 3 - 11% [23]. From the gemcitabine database: PS 0 described 13% of patients, PS 1,2 87% of patients. The figures are relatively similar for chemotherapy and radiotherapy. In the Copenhagen/Manchester study described by Anderson et al. with weekly gemcitabine, 31% of patients improved in performance status defined by at least 4 consecutive observations with scores better than baseline over a period of at least 28 days [24]. In the radiotherapy study the criterion for improvement could be based on just one assessment [23]. Obviously, patients who started with a performance status of zero do not have the potential to improve and therefore are not "eligible" for assessment. When all 4 single-agent gemcitabine non-small cell studies were pooled, there was improvement in performance score from level 2 in 52% of patients (although only 23 patients out of the total group had a PS of 2 initially), which approximated to the 45% improvement of patients with grade 3 (equivalent to PS 2) or worse physical activity as defined in the palliative radiotherapy study [23]. A possible surrogate for performance status change is the effect of chemotherapy on weight: with gemcitabine 67% of patients had a stable weight during the study and 4% an increase - and this was not due to accumulation of fluid in a third space. Clearly the performance status of patients treated with gemcitabine does not always deteriorate and can indeed improve quite markedly in a proportion of patients.

Symptom Relief

Only a few studies have described improvement in disease-related symptoms such as breathlessness etc. [17,18,25]. In the gemcitabine studies an attempt was made to determine the relief or otherwise of disease-related symptoms. Comparison with palliative radiotherapy or other chemotherapy regimens which have documented symptom relief is of course difficult. Relief of specific symptoms by radiotherapy alone, 2 combination chemotherapy

Table 3. Symptom improvement

Treatment	XRT	MVP	PV+M or I	MIP	Gemcitabine	
Reference	MRC '91 [23]	Hardy '89 [25]	Fernandez'89 [26]	Cullen '93 [27]	All studies '93	
					All	Mod/severe
Cough	60%	71%	45%	70%	44%	73%
Haemoptysis	79%	-	91%	92%	63%	100%
Pain	73%	63%	47%	77%	32%	37%
Dyspnoea	61%	65%	78%	46%	26%	51%
Anorexia	67%	-	50%	58%	29%	38%
Response	30%	21%	42%	56%	20%	
Median survival (months)	6	6	NR	9.8	8.1 - 9.2	

XRT - Radiotherapy; PV - cisplatin, vindesine with either M - mitomycin or I - ifosfamide; MVP - mitomycin, vinblastine, cisplatin; MIP - mitomycin, ifosfamide, cisplatin; NR - not recorded
For gemcitabine 'All' refers to the percentage of patients with symptoms (mild, moderate and severe) who had relief; Mod/severe refers to the percentage of patients with just moderate and severe symptoms who improved.
Modified from references 23-27

regimens and single-agent gemcitabine from the pooled database of the 4 studies is described in Table 3 [24-27]. In the gemcitabine studies, for each symptom improvement must have been maintained for at least 4 weeks to be considered clinically relevant. In addition, patients were coded according to the worse symptom experienced between clinic visits, irrespective of the duration of the symptom. Table 3 indicates symptom relief in a good proportion of patients.

It should be noted that in other studies but not those with gemcitabine, e.g. the radiotherapy study, steroids and other symptomatic measures were allowed. The relief of pain with gemcitabine in 32% of the patient group was reflected by a 23% decrease in the use of analgesia. Furthermore, symptom improvement with gemcitabine was more marked for those patients who were classed as having moderate or severe symptoms before treatment (Table 3). The median duration of symptom relief has only been described in the radiotherapy study which approximated to half of the median survival time, i.e., 3 months. From the gemcitabine database the duration of improvement was somewhat more variable for specific symptoms: for example for anorexia and haemoptysis marked relief was obtained for a median of 2-3 months. Dyspnoea and cough was eased over a median of 3-4 months and the median duration of chest pain relief was 5 months. In 2 of the gemcitabine studies of 245 patients any subsequent radiotherapy was recorded. In this patient group only 30% of patients required palliative radiotherapy later.

It is also important to note that patients' and doctors' attitudes to treatment often differ markedly. A study was performed on treatment preferences of patients with cancer in Britain compared with those of radiotherapists and medical oncologists. Out of the one hundred patients who were about to receive chemotherapy and completed questionnaires, 41 had lung cancer. The results are shown in Table 4. Intensive chemotherapy was described as having a considerable number of side-effects such as severe nausea and vomiting, hair loss, frequent use of needles and drips, frequent tiredness, weakness and admission to hospital for 3 or 4 days a month. The mild chemotherapy regimen was described as having fewer side-effects and drawbacks, for

Table 4. Attitude to chemotherapy

Chemotherapy type	Radiotherapist	Oncologist	Patients
	Chance of Cure (1%)		
Intensive	4.5%	20%	53%
Mild	27.3%	51.7%	67%
	Chance of prolonging life (>3 months)		
Intensive	0	10.2%	42.1%
Mild	12.6%	45.0%	53.0%
	Chance of symptom relief (1%)		
Intensive	0	6.8%	42.6%
Mild	2.3%	11.7%	58.7%

Modified from reference 28

example only the occasional use of needles and admission to hospital about once a month. As is shown in Table 4, minimal benefit would make the treatment acceptable to a considerable percentage of patients. Substantial differences are shown between the cancer patients and doctors, indeed patients with cancer are much more likely to accept intensive treatments for a potentially small benefit. Medical oncologists were more likely to accept radical treatment than radiotherapists. After completing 3 months of chemotherapy the responses were again compared on a repeat questionnaire with negligible change. The fact that patients with cancer are much more likely to accept radical intensive treatment with minimal chance of benefit should be borne in mind by medical staff. Treatment options should be presented to patients without prejudging what they will or will not accept [28].

Conclusion

Combination chemotherapy and single-agent therapy with gemcitabine produce an important improvement in performance status in patients with advanced non-small cell lung cancer.

Symptom relief, with single-agent gemcitabine, of distressing cough, haemoptyses and dyspnoea is obtained in over 50% of patients and is of comparable magnitude to that achieved with pallative radiotherapy or combination chemotherapy. Pain is also improved, with a corresponding decrease in analgesia use and lessened anorexia. These improvements were obtained with gemcitabine without the use of supportive measures such as steroids. As the objective response rate confirmed by outside review was 20%, it is obvious that many additional "non-responding" patients obtained symptom relief.

The toxicity spectrum of gemcitabine is favourable. The main haematological toxicity is neutropenia with very little thrombocytopenia, which could be ameliorated by haemopoietic colony stimulating factors. Alopecia is very rare and the main side-effects of lethargy, myalgia and occasional rashes may be relieved with low-dose prednisolone or non-steroidal anti-inflammatory drugs. In the future gemcitabine could be used as a single agent or in combinations in the treatment of stage IV non-small cell lung cancer. In locally advanced non-small cell lung cancer gemcitabine should be studied in combination chemotherapy and with the other modalities of radiotherapy and surgery.

REFERENCES

1   Bakowski M and Crouch JC: Chemotherapy of non-small cell lung cancer: a reappraisal and a look to the future. Cancer Treat Rev 1983 (10):159-172

2   Splinter TAW: Response rate as criterium to evaluate chemotherapy in non-small cell lung cancer. Lung Cancer 1991 (7):91-104

3   Cellerino R, Tummarello D and Piga A: Chemotherapy or not in advanced non-small cell lung cancer? Lung Cancer 1990 (6):99-109

4   Bonomi PD, Finkelstein DM, Ruckdeschel JC et al: Combination chemotherapy versus single agents followed by combination chemotherapy in stage IV non-small-cell lung cancer. A study of the Eastern Cooperative Oncology Group. J Clin Oncol 1989 (7):1602-1613

5   Durrant KR, Berry RJ, Ellis F et al: Comparison of treatment policies in inoperable bronchial carcinoma. Lancet 1971 (1):715-719

6   Laing AH, Berry RJ, Newman CR, Peto J: Treatment of inoperable carcinoma of bronchus. Lancet 1975 (2):1161-1164

7   Rapp E, Pater JL, Willan A et al: Chemotherapy can prolong survival in patients with advanced non small cell lung cancer - report of a Canadian multicenter randomised trial. J Clin Oncol 1988 (6):633-641

8   Klastersky J, Nemec J: Chemotherapy for locally advanced (Stage III) non-small cell lung cancer. Lung Cancer 1991 (7):105-111

9   Buccheri G, Ferrigno D, Rosso A, Vola F: Further evidence in favour of chemotherapy for inoperable non-small cell lung cancer. Lung Cancer 1990 (6):87-98

10 Leung WT, Shiu WCT, Pang JCK et al: Combined chemotherapy and radiotherapy versus best supportive care in the treatment of inoperable non-small cell lung cancer. Oncology 1992 (49):321-326

11 Bunn PA: Future directions in the management of non-small cell lung cancer. Lung Cancer 1993 (9 suppl 2):91-107

12 Evans WK: Rationale for the treatmnt on non-small cell lung cancer. Lung cancer 1993 (9 suppl 2):5-14

13 Cartei G, Cartei F, Cantone A et al: Cisplatin - cyclophosphamide - mitomycin combination chemotherapy with supportive care versus supportive care alone for treatment of metastatic non-small cell lung cancer. JNCI 1993 (85):794-800

14 Jaakkimainen L, Goodwin PJ, Pater J et al: Counting the costs of chemotherapy in a National Cancer Institute of Canada randomised trial in non-small cell lung cancer. J Clin Oncol 1990 (8):1301-1309

15 Souquet PJ, Chauvin F, Boissel JP et al: Polychemotherapy in advanced non-small cell lung cancer: a meta-analysis. Lancet 1993 (342):19-21

16 Bakker W, Van Oosterom AT, Aaronson NK et al: Vindesine, cisplatin and bleomycin combination chemotherapy in non-small cell lung cancer: survival and quality of life. Eur J Cancer Clin Oncol 1986 (22):963-970

17 Thatcher N, Anderson H, Smith DB et al: Ifosfamide by bolus as treatment for advanced non-small cell lung cancer. Cancer Chemother Pharmacol 1986 (18 suppl 2):S30-S34

18 Thatcher N, Smith DB, Lind MJ et al: Double alkylating agent therapy with ifosfamide and cyclophosphamide for advanced non-small cell lung cancer. Cancer 1988 (61):14-18

19 Cullen MH, Joshi R, Chetiyawardana AD, Woodroffe CM: Mitomycin, ifosfamide and cisplatin in non small cell lung cancer: treatment good enough to compare. Br J Cancer 1988 (58):359-361

20 Kris MG, Gralla RJ, Potanovich LM et al: Assessment of pretreatment symptoms and improvement after EDAM + mitomycin + vinblastine (EMV) in patients (pts) with inoperable non-small cell lung cancer (NSCLC). Proc Am Soc Clin Oncol 1990 (9):229, Abst No 883

21 Gurney H, de Campos ES, Dodwell D et al: Ifosfamide and mitomycin in combination for the treatment of patients with progressive advanced non-small cell lung cancer. Eur J Cancer 1991 (27):565-568

22 von Rohr A, Anderson A, McIntosh R, Thatcher N: Phase II study with mitomycin, ifosfamide and carboplatin in inoperable non-small cell lung cancer. Eur J Cancer 1991 (27):1106-1108

23 Medical Research Council by its Lung Cancer Working Party: Inoperable non-small cell lung cancer (NSCLC): a Medical Research Council randomised trial of palliative radiotherapy with two fractions or ten fractions. Br J Cancer 1991 (63):265-270

24 Anderson H, Lund B, Bach F et al: A phase II study of weekly gemcitabine in advanced non-small cell lung cancer. (submitted)

25 Hardy JR, Noble T, Smith IE: Symptom relief with moderate dose chemotherapy (mitomycin C, vinblastine and cisplatin) in advanced non-small cell lung cancer. Br J Cancer 1989 (60):764-766

26 Fernandez C, Rosell R, Abad-Esteve A et al: Quality of life during chemotherapy in non-small cell lung cancer patients. Acta Oncol 1989 (28):29-33

27 Cullen MH: The MIC regimen in non-small cell lung cancer. Lung Cancer 1993 (9 suppl 2):81-89

28 Slevin ML, Stubbs L, Plant HJ et al: Attitude to chemotherapy: comparing views of patients with cancer with those of doctors, nurses and general public. Br Med J 1990 (300):1458-1460

Safety Profile of Gemcitabine, Fludarabine and Cladribine

Maurizio Tonato and Anna Maria Mosconi

Divisione di Oncologia Medica, Policlinico Monteluce, 06122 Perugia, Italy

Antimetabolites are extensively used to treat a variety of tumours. These agents substitute for structurally similar substrates and interfere with important biochemical reactions. The safety profile of recently developed compounds such as gemcitabine, fludarabine and cladribine is discussed in this chapter.

Gemcitabine

In phase I studies the toxicity of gemcitabine was shown to be schedule dependent. Four dosing schedules were evaluated. In the two schedules in which the drug was given more frequently, non-haematological toxicity was a problem: fever, flu-like symptoms and severe hypotension with the daily x 5 q 3 week schedule [1]; fatigue, fever, flu-like symptoms and skin rash with the twice weekly x 6 q 4 week schedule [2]. Using a once every week schedule, gemcitabine was well tolerated, but preclinical data suggest that more frequent administration would be required for maximal activity [4]. A weekly schedule for 3 weeks followed by a week of rest showed minimal non-haematological toxicity and the maximum tolerated dose (MTD) identified in previously treated patients was 790 mg/m^2 with myelotoxicity (thrombocytopenia) being the dose limiting factor [5]. Based on the phase I data, this schedule was the one adopted for the early phase II studies [6,7].

This review summarises the safety data for the phase II studies in which gemcitabine was administered as a 30-minute infusion once a week for 3 weeks followed by a week of rest [8]. The WHO toxicity gradings have been used to report the most severe toxicity experienced by the patient for all courses of drug received.

WHO Laboratory Toxicity

Maximum WHO laboratory toxicity is reported for 790 patients on therapy.

Haemoglobin : WHO grade 3 and 4 toxicity was reported in 6.4% and 0.9% of patients, respectively. In only 2 of 790 patients (0.3%) treatment was discontinued due to anaemia. There was no evidence of cumulative toxicity in the later cycles of gemcitabine treatment. Overall, anaemia was not considered to be a significant problem and was manageable with the use of conventional transfusions, which were required in 19% of patients.

Leukocytes and granulocytes : WHO grade 3 and 4 leukocyte toxicity was recorded in 8.1% and 0.5% of patients, respectively. In only 1 of 790 patients (0.1%) treatment was discontinued due to leukopenia. Previous exposure to cytotoxic chemotherapy appeared to enhance the frequency and severity of leukopenia caused by gemcitabine, although even in previously treated patients leukopenia was rarely dose limiting. Generally, leukocyte depression was manifest by day 7 of each cycle, maximal by day 15-22, and returned to pretreatment levels by day 28. Counts of segmented neutrophils were converted to WHO toxicity scores using criteria for granulocyte toxicity. WHO grade 3 and 4 segmented neutrophil toxicity was 18.7% and 5.7%. The incidence of infection associated with this level of neutropenia was low (grade 2 and above infections were reported in 1.6% and 1.3% of chemotherapy-naive and pretreated patients, respectively). There was no evidence of cumulative toxicity.

Platelets : WHO grade 3 and 4 toxicity was recorded in only 3.7% and 1.0% of patients. In only 3 of 790 patients (0.4%) treatment was discontinued due to thrombocytopenia. There was no evidence of cumulative toxicity. Patients previously treated with cytotoxic chemotherapy tended to show more pronounced platelet toxicity. There appeared to be no difference in toxicity between patients starting at the 800, 1000 and 1250 mg/m^2 dose levels.

ALT, AST, alkaline phosphatase, bilirubin : WHO grade 3 and 4 toxicity was as follows: ALT 7.4% and 1.8%; AST 5.7% and 1.4%; alkaline phosphatase 4.5% and 2.1%; bilirubin 1.0% and 0.5%. In only 4 of 790 patients (0.5%) treatment was discontinued due to abnormalities in liver function (1 of these patients had a history of chronic alcoholism). There was no increase in the median distribution of maximum values across cycles for alkaline phosphatase or bilirubin. Levels of transaminases did not increase beyond cycles 1 and 2, suggesting that there is no cumulative toxicity.

Blood urea nitrogen, creatinine, proteinuria, haematuria : WHO grade 3 toxicity for each of these parameters was 0, 0.1%, 0.5% and 1.3%, respectively. No WHO grade 4 toxicity was recorded. Three of 790 patients (0.4%) experienced renal failure whilst on gemcitabine therapy. Overall, mild proteinuria and haematuria were commonly reported but these were rarely clinically significant. Renal toxicity as assessed by BUN and serum creatinine was not a significant problem; the disproportionate rise in BUN values relative to creatinine suggested a prerenal component.

Overall, these laboratory abnormalities were usually mild, easily reversible and rarely dose limiting.

In a safety overview including 1,598 patients, 5 patients were reported to develop haemolytic uraemic syndrome [9].

WHO Symptomatic Toxicity

WHO symptomatic toxicities are reported for a subset of 439 patients.

Nausea and vomiting : WHO grade 3 and 4 was recorded in 19.8% and 0.9% of patients. In only 0.9% of patients treatment was discontinued due to nausea and vomiting. Overall, nausea and vomiting required therapy in about 20% of patients, were rarely dose limiting and were easily manageable with standard antiemetics; 5-HT$_3$ antiemetics were usually not required.

Oral toxicity : WHO grade 3 and 4 toxicity was 0.2% and 0%. In only 1 of 439 patients treatment was discontinued due to oral toxicity.

Diarrhoea : WHO grade 3 and 4 toxicity was 0.5% and 0% and in no patient treatment was discontinued due to diarrhoea.

Pulmonary toxicity : WHO grade 3 and 4 toxicity was 1.6% and 0.2%, respectively. Although drug-related dyspnoea was commonly reported, it was usually mild and rarely required specific therapy. Whether dyspnoea is actually related to the administration of gemcitabine or to underlying cardiac or pulmonary dysfunction is still unclear. For most of these patients alternative aetiologies were identified, e.g. pleural effusions, pneumonia, atelectasis, pericardial effusions.

However, 3 patients were reported to develop severe dyspnoea: in two of them grade 3 dyspnoea requiring hospitalisation occurred 1-2 hours after the administration of gemcitabine and resolved 4-5 hours later [10]. Treatment was discontinued in both patients; no other manifestations of allergy were found. The third patient died of respiratory failure several hours after the second dose of gemcitabine [11]. In any case, investigators should be aware of the possibility of dyspnoea and bronchospasm developing shortly after the administration of gemcitabine, particularly in patients with pre-existing pulmonary disease.

Fever : WHO grade 3 and 4 fever was 0.7% and 0%. Fever was frequently associated with other flu-like symptoms which will be discussed later. Fever was usually mild, of brief duration, easily manageable and rarely dose limiting.

Allergic toxicity : WHO grade 3 and 4 was 0.2% and 0%.

Cutaneous toxicity : WHO grade 3 and 4 toxicity was 0.2% and 0%. A transient, mild erythematous pruritic rash was reported; it sometimes subsided or improved despite discontinuation of therapy. Desquamation was observed on at least one occasion. In only 2 of 439 patients treatment was discontinued due to cutaneous toxicity.

Hair toxicity : WHO grade 3 and 4 was 0.5% and 0%. Overall, there was little hair toxicity and 86.7% of patients had no hair loss at all.

Infection toxicity : WHO grade 3 and 4 was 0.9% and 0.2%. In only 2 patients treatment was discontinued due to severe infection associated with leukopenia. Neither the starting dose nor the previous chemotherapy status of the patient had an effect on either the frequency or severity of the infection episodes. Overall, drug-related infection was usually mild, rarely dose limiting and easily manageable.

Cardiac rhythm, cardiac function, pericarditis : WHO grade 3 and 4 toxicity was as follows: cardiac rhythm 0.2% and 0%; cardiac function 0.7% and 0.2%; pericarditis 0% and 0%. Overall, there is no evidence that gemcitabine causes cardiac toxicity.

State of consciousness : WHO grade 3 and 4 toxicity was 0.5% and 0%. Variable central nervous system symptoms were reported: somnolence, agitation, insomnia, dizziness, paraesthesia, confusion, convulsion, coma.

Peripheral neurotoxicity, constipation : There was no WHO grade 3 or 4 peripheral neurotoxicity. WHO grade 1 and 2 was 3.2% and 0.2%, respectively. WHO grade 3 and 4 constipation was 0.2% and 0%.

Pain : WHO grade 3 and 4 pain was 1.1% and 0%.

Adverse Events not Covered by the WHO Toxicity Gradings

Certain events are not covered by the WHO grading system and were recorded separately. These are summarised for 790 patients on therapy.

Flu-like symptoms : The total number of patients with flu-like symptoms was 155 (19.6%), but only in 1 patient treatment was discontinued due to this side-effect. Headache, back pain, chills, myalgia, asthenia and anorexia were the most commonly reported symptoms. Myalgia was generally considered to be drug related even when reported as an isolated symptom. Cough, rhinitis, malaise and insomnia were also reported. Flu-like symptoms might also have accounted for some, but not all, cases of fever. The flu-like symptoms were usually mild, of brief duration (often on the day of treatment only) and rarely dose limiting. The mechanism of this event is unknown. Investigators have reported that symptoms can be relieved with paracetamol.

Oedema : Oedema of any type was seen in 28.4% of patients, and was classified as mild in 13.5%, moderate in 12.1%, and severe in 2.6% of patients. In 6 out of 790 patients (0.8%) treatment was discontinued due to oedema. Oedema is not associated with any evidence of cardiac, hepatic or renal failure; this suggests a vasculitic effect and a capillary leak syndrome as possible cause of the oedema.

Overall, the safety data demonstrate that gemcitabine has a favourable side-effect profile. One of the features which make gemcitabine unusual is the low incidence of the adverse events, namely myelosuppression, nausea, vomiting and alopecia, that are usually associated with cytotoxic drugs. This non-overlapping toxicity makes the drug an attractive candidate for trial in combination with other cytotoxic agents.

Fludarabine

A wide variety of doses and schedules of administration of fludarabine have been evaluated in phase I trials [12].

Myelosuppression was the dose-limiting toxicity with all schedules used, with leukopenia being more prominent than thrombocytopenia. One aspect of the leukopenia noted in one study was the profound decrease in lymphocyte counts [13]; it was documented in the patients of this trial that fludarabine was lymphocytotoxic, with the greatest cytotoxicity towards T lymphocytes [14].

A severe neurotoxicity [15] was reported in patients with acute leukaemia receiving high-dose fludarabine ($\geq$ 96 mg/m^2/day for 5-7 days). Thirteen of 36 patients developed this toxicity 21 to 60 days after receiving the last course of fludarabine. The toxicity developed in patients on both bolus and continuous infusion. Neurotoxicity usually was present as visual deficits followed by progressive deterioration of mental status, coma, and death. No specific examinations such as cerebrospinal fluid, electroencephalogram, computerised axial tomography scans, or nuclear magnetic resonance scans were helpful. No predisposing conditions (e.g. prior brain irradiation) were identified. Findings at autopsy in 3 patients showed a diffuse demyelation in the brain and spinal cord, particularly in the occipital cortex around the optic tracts.

Other toxicities noted in phase I trials included mild to moderate nausea and vomiting, and a rare and reversible interstitial pneumonitis [16].

Because of side-effects observed in phase I trials, the dose and schedule of fludarabine were modified to reduce toxicity while still retaining clinical effectiveness. The most widely used schedule in phase II trials has been 20-30 mg/m2 daily intravenous infusion for 5 consecutive days, with the course repeated monthly. Myelotoxicity becomes excessive at higher doses (>30 mg/m2 daily for 5 days), whereas the drug may not be sufficiently active at doses <15 mg/m2.

Consequently, 20 to 30 mg/m2 administered as a 30-minute infusion daily for 5 days remains the recommended schedule of drug administration. At these recommended doses the drug has been well tolerated and adverse events have generally been mild to moderate [17,18], even if clinical experience with fludarabine is still relatively limited and toxicity data based on larger patient populations are necessary.

Reversible bone marrow suppression, predominantly granulocytopenia, is the dose-limiting toxicity reported with fludarabine. Treatment of 133 patients with chronic lymphocytic leukaemia (CLL) was associated with severe neutropenia (<500/µl) in 59% of patients. Haemoglobin decreased by 20 g/l from baseline in 60% of patients, and platelet count fell to less than 50% of baseline in 55% of patients [19]. Myelosuppression did not appear to be cumulative according to 2 studies in patients with CLL [20,21]. In a study of 25 patients treated for non-Hodgkin lymphomas (NHL), however, the myelosuppression appeared to be cumulative in patients receiving 3 or more courses [22].

Non-haematological toxicity data from 101 patients with CLL who received fludarabine in the MD Anderson Cancer Studies have been summarised (US Prescribing Information Fludarabine, Berlex Laboratories, 1992): mild to moderate nausea and vomiting (36%), fever (60%), pain (20%), infection (33%), diarrhoea and skin rash (about 18%) were the most commonly reported adverse events.

A relatively high incidence of fever or infection, occurring in 62% of patients with NHL [23], as well as opportunistic infections [24] was reported. This may be due to depletion of CD4+ cells during fludarabine therapy [25]. Depletion of CD4+ cells was also associated with an increased incidence of listeriosis in patients receiving fludarabine in combination with prednisone [26].

It has been reported that a few patients had reversible interstitial pulmonary infiltrates thought to represent pulmonary toxicity [27-29]. All patients responded to corticosteroid treatment. In one instance, however, respiratory support and discontinuation of fludarabine therapy was required [29].

Tumour lysis syndrome occurred in several cases [30]; this responded well to conventional treatment and did not recur in subsequent courses when fludarabine was administered with allopurinol, forced diuresis, and alkalinisation of the urine. Patients at high risk of developing a tumour lysis syndrome are those with massive lymphadenopathy, splenomegaly, and lymphocytosis ≥200.000/µl.

Three cases of severe autoimmune haemolytic anaemia possibly associated with fludarabine administration were observed [31,32]. One case occurred 5 weeks after receiving the last course of fludarabine, a second case did not recur in spite of treatment continuation, and both patients had a prior history of haemolytic anaemia which occurs in 10-25% of patients with CLL.

To date, with the recommended doses there has been only 1 well-documented case of severe neurotoxicity encountered at the higher doses (≥96 mg/m2/day for 5-7 days) in phase I trials. This occurred in a 66-year-old man with mycosis fungoides receiving fludarabine 18 to 22.5 mg/m2/day for 5 days for only 3 courses [33]. Autopsy revealed CNS involvement of mycosis fungoides as well as multifocal demyelation. However, the localisation of mycosis fungoides in the brain might have allowed greater drug penetration and hence neurotoxicity at a much lower dose.

The occurrence of neurotoxicity appears to be related to peak plasma levels of fludarabine, since no other incidents have been seen in patients who received repeated low doses of the drug with a cumulative dose equivalent or higher than those attained with high-dose schedules.

Six of 62 patients (10%) with NHL developed grade 3 neurological toxicity on receiving fludarabine 18 mg/m2/day for 5 days. The toxicity included reversible visual changes, auditory hallucinations, confusion and fatigue; fludarabine was discontinued in all cases [34]. Recently, reversible neurotoxicity was reported in 1 patient with mycosis fungoides and in 1 patient with CLL [35].

The irreversible neurotoxicity seen in phase I studies with high doses makes fludarabine a poor candidate for high-dose chemotherapy regimens, which would require either bone marrow or peripheral blood stem cell support.

The kidney is the primary route of excretion of fludarabine and limited data suggest that excessive toxicity may be encountered in patients with renal dysfunction. Dosage reduction should be considered in patients with creatinine clearance $\leq$ 3 l/h (50 ml/min).

Other patients at increased risk of fludarabine toxicity are elderly patients and patients with bone marrow impairment.

Cladribine (2-chlorodeoxyadenosine)

In phase I studies cladribine (2-chlorodeoxyadenosine, 2-CDA), given as a continuous intravenous infusion usually over 7 days, was essentially non-toxic, apart from bone marrow suppression [36,37].

Since the drug has pronounced anti-leukaemic activity, it was used in the preparation of leukaemia patients for bone marrow transplantation. In these patients doses higher than 0.26 mg/kg per day for 10-14 days caused renal and central nervous system toxicity [38]. The adverse events were so severe that some patients required haemodialysis; the renal toxicity was reversible in those patients who survived the other complications of bone marrow transplantation.

Such toxicity never manifested itself at doses of 0.1 mg/kg/day given as a continuous intravenous infusion for 7 days; this is the optimal and most widely used schedule [39].

In one study which summarised the experience with 80 patients receiving 2-CDA on a standard schedule, myelosuppression (25%) and infection (43%) were the most important adverse effects [40].

Neutropenia to over 50% of the initial value occurred in 46% of patients, thrombocytopenia in 8%, and lymphopenia <0.5 x 10⁹/l was seen in 41% of patients. Lymphopenia at the start of

treatment and on day 14 was associated with a higher risk of severe infections. Almost two-thirds of all infection episodes were opportunistic, all of them starting within 4 weeks from the initiation of therapy; in 6.3% of patients the infection was fatal.

2-CDA typically causes protracted severe lymphopenia with a marked decrease in the CD4 to CD8 ratio lasting 6 to 9 months after treatment; the drug-induced immunosuppression might lead to such a high incidence of infectious complications. Nevertheless, a survey of the literature on 520 patients treated with 2-CDA [40] shows a low rate of infectious complications (about 15%).

The higher incidence of infections in the above-mentioned study may be due to the inclusion of many patients with advanced stage of disease and heavily pretreated. Similar data are confirmed by recent experiences [41,42].

In patients with particularly severe lymphopenia at the start of therapy the value of prophylactic anti-infective therapy should be investigated.

Infection caused by *Listeria monocytogenes* has been described in a patient with CLL who had received fludarabine until 5 weeks before 2-CDA administration [43]. Since the risk of listeriosis seems to be associated only with the combined use of fludarabine and corticosteroids [26], the patient's susceptibility to listeria infection may be due to treatment with 2-CDA alone or to the sequential use of fludarabine and 2-CDA.

When repeated courses of 2-CDA were given, as in the treatment of CLL or lymphomas, thrombocytopenia was reported to become the limiting toxicity in 20-30% of patients [41,42].

Erythroid macrocytosis was often observed in patients who had received as many as 6 courses of 2-CDA; this condition persisted for 6 months or more after the last course of the drug. Fever was reported in about one third of patients with hairy cell leukaemia; because cultures were almost always negative in these patients the fever was probably related to cytokine release.

A few cases of intracerebral haemorrhages were reported [40,42]; in some of these, severe thrombocytopenia was documented [42].

Other toxic effects were reported only rarely [40]: mild nausea without vomiting (8%), mucositis (4%), and phlebitis at the site of infusion (8%). No clinically significant hair loss or any other tissue dysfunction was observed. There has been no increased frequency of second tumours; however, since the compound is incorporated into DNA, it is likely that it is mutagenic [44].

REFERENCES

1   O'Rourke T, Brown T, Havlin T et al: Phase I clinical trial of difluorodeoxycytidine (Ly188011) given as an intravenous bolus on five consecutive days. Proc Am Assoc Cancer Res 1989 (30):82 (abstr)
2   Poplin E, Redman B, Flaherty L et al: Difluorodeoxycytidine (dFdC): A phase I study. Proc Am Soc Oncol 1989 (30):282 (abstr)
3   Vermorken J, Guastalla JP, Hatty SR et al: Phase I study of gemcitabine using a once every 2 week schedule. Eur J Cancer 1994 (submitted)
4   Grindey GB, Hertel LW, Plunkett W: Cytotoxicity and antitumor effect of 2',2'-difluorodeoxycytidine (gemcitabine). Cancer Invest 1990 (2):313
5   Abbruzzese JL, Grunewald R, Weeks EA et al: A phase I clinical, plasma and cellular pharmacology study of gemcitabine. J Clin Oncol 1991 (9):491-498
6   Anderson H, Lund B, Hansen H et al: Phase II study of gemcitabine in patients with advanced colorectal cancer. Proc Am Soc Clin Oncol 1991 (10):848 (abstr)
7   Abbruzzese JL, Pazdur R, Ajani J et al: A phase II trial of gemcitabine in patients with advanced colorectal cancer. Proc Am Soc Clin Oncol 1991 (10):456 (abstr)
8   Tonato M: Gemcitabine safety overview. Satellite symposium of the 7th European Conference on Clinical Oncology and Cancer Nursing. Jerusalem 1993 pp 14-16
9   Ely Lilly, data on file
10   Mertens WC, Eisenhauer EA, Moore M et al: Gemcitabine in advanced renal cell carcinoma. Ann Oncol 1993 (4):331-332
11   Eisenhauer E, Cormier Y, Gregg R et al: Gemcitabine is active in patients with previously untreated extensive small cell lung cancer. A phase II study of the National Cancer Institute of Canada Clinical Trials Group. Proc Am Soc Clin Oncol 1992 (11):309 (abstr)
12   Von Hoff DD: Phase I clinical trials with fludarabine phosphate. Sem Oncol 1990 (17 suppl 8):33-38
13   Hutton JJ, Von Hoff DD, Kuhn J et al: Phase I clinical investigation of 9-ß-D-arabinofuranosyl-2-fluoroadenine 5'-monophosphate (NSC 312887), a new purine antimetabolite. Cancer Res 1984 (44):4183-4186
14   Bolt DH, Von Hoff DD, Kuhn JG et al: Effects on human peripheral lymphocytes of in vivo administration of 9-ß-D-arabinofuranosyl-2-fluoroadenine-5'-monophosphate (NSC 312887), a new purine antimetabolite. Cancer Res 1984 (44):4661-4666
15   Chun HG, Leyland Jones BR, Caryk SM et al: Central nervous system toxicity of fludarabine phosphate. Cancer Treat Rep 1986 (70):1225-1228
16   Hurst PG, Habib MP, Garewal H et al: Pulmonary toxicity associated with fludarabine monophosphate. Invest New Drugs 1987 (5):207-210
17   Cheson BD: Issues for the future. Development of fludarabine phosphate. Sem Oncol 1990 (17 suppl 8):71-78
18   Cheson BD: New antimetabolites in the treatment of human malignancies. Sem Oncol 1992 (19):695-706
19   Ross SR, Mc Tavish D, Faulds D: Fludarabine. A review of its pharmacological properties and therapeutic potential in malignancy. Drugs 1993 (45):737-759
20   Keating MJ, Kantarjian H, Talpaz M et al: Fludarabine: a new agent with major activity against chronic lymphocytic leukemia. Blood 1989 (74):19-25
21   Keating MJ, Kantarjian H, O'Brien S et al: Fludarabine: a new agent with marked cytoreductive activity in untreated chronic lymphocytic leukemia. J Clin Oncol 1991 (9):44-49
22   Leiby JM, Snider KM, Kraut EH et al: Phase II trial of 9-ß-D-arabinofuranosyl-2-fluoroadenine-5'-monophosphate in non-Hodgkin's lymphoma: prospective comparison of response with deoxycytidine kinase activity. Cancer Res 1987 (47): 2719-2722
23   Redman JR, Cabanillas F, Velasquez WS et al: Phase II trial of fludarabine phosphate in lymphoma: an effective new agent in low-grade lymphoma. J Clin Oncol 1992 (10):790-794
24   Sanders C, Perez EA, Lawrence HJ: Opportunistic infections in patients with chronic lymphocytic leukemia following treatment with fludarabine. Correspondence. Am J Hematol 1992 (39):314-315
25   Wijermans et al: Proc Am Soc Hematol 1992, abstr 174
26   Anaissie E, Kontoyiannis DP, Kantarjian H et al: Listeriosis in patients with chronic lymphocytic leukemia who were treated with fludarabine and prednisone. Ann Intern Med 1990 (117):466-469
27   Cervantes F, Saldago C, Montserrat E et al: Fludarabine for prolymphocytic leukemia and risk of interstitial pneumonitis. Lancet 1990 (336):1130
28   Hurst PG, Habib MP, Garewal H et al: Pulmonary toxicity associated with fludarabine monophosphate. Invest New Drugs 1987 (5):207-210
29   Kane GC, McMichael AJ, Patrick H et al: Pulmonary toxicity and acute respiratory failure associated with fludarabine monophosphate. Respir Med 1992 (86):261-263
30   List AF, Kummet TD, Adams JD et al: Tumor lysis syndrome complicating treatment of chronic lymphocytic leukemia with fludarabine phosphate. Am J Med 1990 (89):388-390
31   Bastion Y, Coiffier B, Dumontet C et al: Severe autoimmune hemolytic anemia in two patients treated with fludarabine for chronic lymphocytic leukemia. Ann Oncol 1992 (3):171-173
32   Tosti S, Caruso R, D'Adamo F et al: Severe autoimmune hemolytic anemia in a patient with chronic lymphocytic leukemia responsive to fludarabine-based treatment. Ann Haemat 1992 (65):238-239
33   Merkel DE, Griffin NL, Kaga-Hallet K et al: Central nervous system toxicity of fludarabine. Cancer Treat Rep 1986 (70):1449-1450

34 Hocster HS, Kim K, Green MD et al: Activity of fludarabine in previously treated non-Hodgkin's low-grade lymphoma: results of an Eastern Cooperative Oncology Group study. J Clin Oncol 1992 (10):28-32

35 Cohen RB, Abdallah JM, Gray JR et al: Reversible neurologic toxicity in patients treated with standard-dose fludarabine phosphate for mycosis fungoides and chronic lymphocytic leukemia. Ann Intern Med 1993 (118):114-116

36 Carson DA, Wasson DB, Beutler E et al: Antileukemic and immunosuppressive activity of 2-chloro-2'-deoxyadenosine. Proc Natl Acad Sci USA 1984 (81):2232-2236

37 Carson DA, Wasson DB, Lamon J et al: A potent new anti-lymphocyte agent: 2-chlorodeoxyadenosine. Blood 1982 (60 suppl 1):161a

38 Beutler E, Piro LD, Savan A et al: 2-chlorodeoxyadenosine (2-CdA): a potent chemotherapeutic and immunosuppressive nucleoside. Leukemia Lymphoma 1991 (5):1-8

39 Beutler E: Cladribine (2-chlorodeoxyadenosine). Lancet 1992 (340):952-956

40 Betticher DC, Fey MF, Von Rohr A et al: High incidence of infections after 2-chlorodeoxyadenosine (2-CdA) therapy in patients with malignant lymphomas and chronic and acute leukemias. Ann Oncol 1994 (5):57-64

41 Juliusson G, Liliemark J: High complete remission rate from 2-chloro-2'-deoxyadenosine in previously treated patients with B cell chronic lymphocytic leukemia: response predicted by rapid decrease of blood lymphocyte count. J Clin Oncol 1993 (11):679-689

42 O'Brien S, Kantarjian H, Estey E et al: Lack of effect of 2-chlorodeoxyadenosine therapy in patients with chronic lymphocytic leukemia refractory to fludarabine therapy. N Engl J Med 1994 (330):319-322

43 Spielberger RT, Stock W, Larson RA: Lysteriosis after 2-chlorodeoxyadenosine treatment. Correspondence. N Engl J Med 1993 (328):813-814

44 Carson DA, Wasson DB, Teatle R et al: Specific toxicity of 2-chlorodeoxyadenosine toward resting and proliferating human lymphocytes. Blood 1983 (62):737-743

If you have any concerns about our products,
you can contact us on
ProductSafety@springernature.com

In case Publisher is established outside the EU,
the EU authorized representative is:
**Springer Nature Customer Service Center GmbH
Europaplatz 3, 69115 Heidelberg, Germany**

Printed by Libri Plureos GmbH
in Hamburg, Germany